Models of Nursing in Practice

Models of Nursing in Practice

A Pattern for Practical Care

Paula McGee

Nursing Research Fellow
Nursing Research Unit
University of Central England
Birmingham, UK

Stanley Thornes (Publishers) Ltd

First published in 1998
by Stanley Thornes (Publishers) Ltd
Ellenborough House
Wellington Street
CHELTENHAM
GL50 1YW
United Kingdom

98 99 00 01 02 / 10 9 8 7 6 5 4 3 2 1

A catalogue record for this book is available from the British Library

ISBN 0-7487-3343-4

Typeset by WestKey Ltd, Falmouth, Cornwall
Printed and bound in Great Britain
by Scotprint Ltd, Musselburgh, Scotland

FOR LAVARCHAM AND PAUL MEEHAN

Contents

Acknowledgements

I wish to thank the very many people who helped and advised me during the development of this book. In particular I wish to thank patients and their families for the opportunities to learn from them; my students and colleagues; Madeleine Stafford for her patience and advice in developing the text.

Introduction $\boxed{1}$

Nursing is about caring for the sick and dying. It is about helping people to achieve independence whilst living with disabilities. It is about helping people to cope with terrifying difficulties. It is about enabling people to manage their own health and much more. Nursing is essentially active and practical. We give nursing care to patients and it is on the performance of that care that our expertise is judged. We are considered to be good nurses because of what we do, not because of what we say about what we do.

In such a performance-related profession, thinking and talking about nursing, generating ideas for practice and theory in general, can be viewed as the work of people who have no ability in the real world of nursing. If this is so, then we do not need to use our brains to nurse. We can, like the proverbial monkey, simply learn our tasks and orders, and ignore the fact that what we do requires considerable knowledge, understanding and skill, all of which have a theoretical framework.

All other practice-orientated disciplines function in this way. Medicine, for example, has rigorous theoretical foundations. A practitioner draws on knowledge from a range of disciplines such as the biological and behavioural sciences and integrates this with the knowledge of medicine. Medical practice is based on a systematic application of knowledge and understanding. This framework or model is evident in the approach of the doctor in examining, diagnosing and treating the patient.

Nurses and allied health disciplines approach their practice in the same way but with different applications. For example, Mr Smith is 'on bed rest' and has awakened this morning to find his bed soaked in urine. This has never happened to him before and he is very upset. When the nurse has finished caring for him, he seems more cheerful and is ready to eat breakfast. In referring to this event, the nurse is likely to say, 'I've just given Mr Smith a little wash and sat him up for breakfast', dismissing what actually took place as if this care, and the way in which it was carried out, was not important to the patient. The nurse will not acknowledge the use of theory in dealing with the situation. Yet theory has been applied: from nursing skills and knowledge to provide practical care; from psychology to help alleviate Mr Smith's distress; from physiology to determine the cause of incontinence and the subsequent care for his skin in preventing soreness; and from microbiology to help prevent the spread of cross infection.

Thus the nurse has integrated knowledge from several different sources and applied them within a framework which enabled that nurse to provide care and the patient to feel cared for. Theory is of direct importance in our practice. We use it a lot more than we might like to think and we certainly need to use it a lot more and more consciously. This means reappraising our ideas about what both theory and nursing are, as well as asking some searching questions about the frameworks that we use.

There is nothing esoteric about a framework or model for our practice. It is simply a way of organizing our knowledge and understanding for the benefit of our patients. We do this every day in the performance of care activities. In giving a bed bath we gather together all that we need and set about it in a systematic fashion which is modified depending on the needs of the patient, the working environment and our own level of skill. We would criticize a nurse who lacked the ability to organize and deliver a simple procedure such as a bed bath; who constantly left the bedside to fetch yet another item that had been forgotten; who neglected elementary factors such as keeping the patient covered.

Having a framework or model for our whole practice is not really any different. It is simply on a larger scale. A framework for our practice requires us to examine our approach to nursing as a whole, in relation to our specific type of patients, within our particular working environment and taking into account the personality of each individual nurse.

This book explores ways of doing this. It is, first of all, for experienced practitioners who know about nursing but it is hoped that those who are new to the profession will also find it helpful. It is particularly aimed at those who question the status quo and who want to develop or formalize their ideas about nursing in their own field of practice. Nurses undertaking diploma or degree modules which examine the apparent gap between practice and theory will find this issue explored in some depth.

The book begins by examining the nature of theory itself and gives examples of the ways in which we use theory in everyday nursing practice, whether we acknowledge it or not. This second chapter also enables the reader to begin weighing up the pros and cons of a theory and determine its usefulness in the practice setting.

Chapter 3 looks at theory in nursing and explores in some depth the so-called gap between theory and practice. An overview of the different strategies which have been employed as solutions to this perceived gap is also provided. In particular this chapter introduces the idea that practitioners can and should develop their own approaches to nursing.

This idea underpins the rest of the book and is approached in two ways. My own thoughts about nursing have gradually evolved through a combination of clinical practice and teaching. Many of the factors which have helped to shape my thinking are discussed here and the final chapter presents my own theory of nursing. This is characterized by an emphasis on practical and interpersonal skills, the nurse as a person and the transcultural elements of nursing care. In developing this theory, I have tried to bear in mind the criticisms outlined above. The McGee theory of nursing is, I hope, jargon free, reasonably easy to understand and practical. The final chapter gives some examples of ways in which it can be applied to patients with different types of problem both in the community and in hospital.

In addition this book encourages you, the reader, to develop your own views about nursing through a series of exercises, discussion topics and reading suggestions. These ask you to set out your thoughts about:

- Patients. For example how would you describe them and what are their particular needs?
- Health. For example what is health and how is it important in caring for your patients?
- The setting in which you work/would like to work when you are qualified. For example do you work in a hospital, a factory or in patients' homes? How does the environment in which you work affect the way you practise nursing?
- Nursing itself. For example how would you describe the nursing that you do? What are the positive aspects of this work and what are the stresses?
- Wider issues related to practice. These include critically examining the points raised by key texts.

Alongside these tasks, each chapter presents ideas from other nurse theorists so that you can compare and contrast your thinking with theirs. You can complete all these exercises working on your own or with a group of colleagues. It is advisable to record both your answers and your developing ideas as you progress through the book in preparation for Chapter 8. This will help you bring the different threads together to construct the first version of your own approach to nursing. Some examples of embryonic theories will be presented and discussed. Finally this chapter will suggest ways in which you and your colleagues might set about implementing your ideas. I hope you will find this book helpful. Feedback and comments would be welcome.

2 | The nature of theory

WHAT IS A THEORY?

In trying to answer this question it is useful to begin by examining some definitions of theory. In doing so we can identify the main components which can be found in any theory, irrespective of the discipline in which it is based.

The structure of a theory

Exercises

> **Exercise 2.1 Definitions of theory**
>
> Look at the following statements. What do they tell us about theory?
>
> 1. 'A theory is a conceptual system or framework invented to some purpose' (Dickoff and James 1968).
> 2. 'A creative and rigorous structuring of ideas that projects a tentative, purposeful and systematic view of phenomena' (Chinn and Kramer 1991).
> 3. 'Theory is a logically consistent set of propositions that presents a systematic view of a phenomenon' (Keck 1989).

The definitions presented in the above exercise convey the information that a theory contains ideas (1); that it has some sort of framework (1) or structure (2) which is 'logically consistent' (3). Theory has a purpose (1) which is to provide a 'systematic view of phenomena' (2). From this we can conclude that a theory is not a single entity.

Ideas and concepts

A theory is made up of a collection of ideas which are grouped together (Fig. 2.1). These groups are called *concepts* and they are themselves linked together (Chinn and Kramer 1995). For example, the concept of caring (Clifford 1995) might incorporate ideas about love, duty and parenting all of which are interlinked. It might also be linked to the concept of nursing which includes ideas about professional conduct, the knowledge base of nurses and so on. Within any theory, some concepts will be very important and others less so.

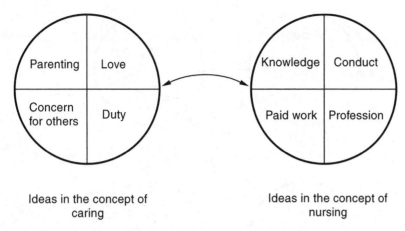

| Parenting | Love |
| Concern for others | Duty |

| Knowledge | Conduct |
| Paid work | Profession |

Ideas in the concept of
caring

Ideas in the concept of
nursing

Fig. 2.1 A theory is a collection of ideas or concepts grouped together to form concepts.

Grouping concepts

The way in which concepts are grouped is not haphazard. These group-ings are systematically organized and logical and should be the result of rigorous testing where possible.

The links between concepts may take several different forms. Figure 2.2 shows some of the possible concepts which might be present in a theory about care of the elderly. In looking at these concepts it might be possible to identify (Fawcett and Downs 1992) the following:

- The *strength* of the links between certain concepts. For example, there may be strong links between the concepts of family, caring and community but weak links between community, poverty and discrimination.
- *Whether one concept gives rise to another.* For example, there is an increased likelihood that in old age individuals will develop a health problem or disability. As a result they may need nursing or community care. Thus if one concept becomes a reality then the others will follow.
- *Whether some concepts are essential.* For example it might be argued that caring is essential to a number of other concepts such as nursing. Without caring, nursing cannot exist.

In relation to these concepts, we also have to consider the research that supported both their development and that of the theory as a whole. Theories differ in terms of how and when data (information) were collected and analysed. This in turn can affect the reliability of the theory.

Clarity and simplicity in theory

The quality of the presentation of the theory is also important. Theory must be communicable if it is to serve any purpose whatsoever (Dickoff and James 1968) but the clarity of the communication can affect the way in which the theory is perceived. Clarity has four dimensions (Chinn and

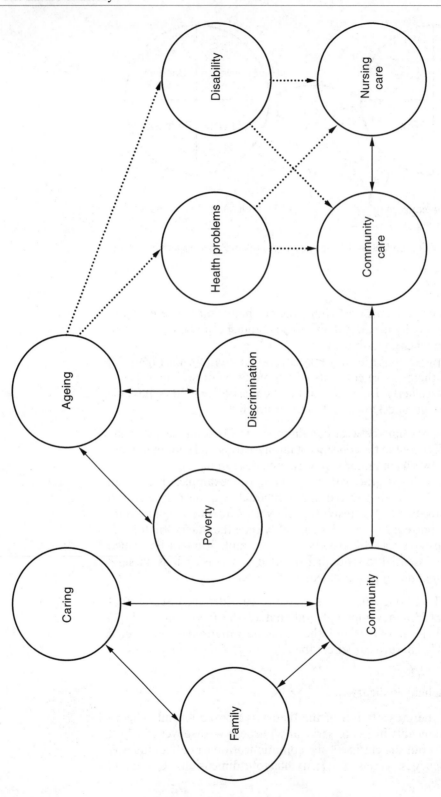

Fig. 2.2 Concepts in a theory about care of the elderly.

Kramer 1995) the first two of which are concerned with language whilst the other two address structure.

Semantic clarity requires that concepts are clearly defined. Terminology must be unambiguous, especially if it is borrowed from other disciplines or is newly coined. Excessive wordage should be avoided. Brief, easily understood examples should be included where appropriate. *Semantic consistency* should be a part of the development of a theory over time, which can take years. The language used in the theory must be consistent throughout so that, even though changes occur, it is still possible to follow what is being said.

Discussion Topic 2.1

Compare and contrast two theories of nursing in terms of how clear and easy they are to understand.

Discussion

Structural clarity refers to the network of ideas used to form each concept and the relationships between concepts themselves. All of this must be clearly explained so that the structure of the theory is apparent. *Structural consistency* requires that the structure of the theory remains clear and consistent as it develops. This is not to say that developing ideas and concepts may not undergo any changes but that the concepts should remain logically interrelated and the structure consistent (Chinn and Kramer 1995). In simple terms the theory should hang together in the paper that you are reading as well as in other publications on the subject by the same author.

Clarity should not be confused with *simplicity*. A theory may be expressed in very clear terms but at the same time demonstrate complex ideas. On the other hand, complicated terms may be used to explain something which is quite simple. This is unhelpful to both the reader and the theorist. Unnecessarily complex language excludes the reader and may even evoke hostility. The theorist's work is then just so much wasted effort because 'if at the end of the day you cannot tell others what you have been doing, then your doing has been in vain' (Schrodinger 1951).

It has to be acknowledged that many nurse theorists unwittingly fall into the trap of presenting their work in an esoteric manner which alienates practitioners. Consequently they end up talking only to one another, reinforcing the image of nursing theory as an elitist pursuit. Nobody likes being made to feel stupid because they cannot understand and so practitioners either ignore theory altogether or denigrate it as meaningless, which in this context is exactly what it is.

Discussion Topic 2.2

Find examples of unnecessarily complex language from other sources, e.g. letters from official sources. What are these examples trying to say? What effect does the language have?

Discussion

Clarity is therefore a crucial element in the communication of theory. Nurses need both the skill and the confidence to challenge jargon, obscure language and verbiage. Only then will the profession begin to identify what elements are truly of use in practice.

WHY DO WE NEED THEORY?

Theories have a practical purpose in helping us understand phenomena, that is aspects of the world around us. Theories range from those which seem to explain only one aspect of a phenomenon to those which explain the whole of it. For example Festinger's theory of cognitive dissonance attempts to explain one aspect of human behaviour whereas Freud's tries to explain the whole of it.

Theories can be divided into three groups (Fawcett 1995). *Grand theories* are broadest in scope, and tend to be abstract in nature. They are more philosophical than other types of theory and therefore may be difficult to test and use in real life. Fawcett (1995) suggests that Leininger's theory of transcultural care is a grand theory because it encompasses every aspect of life. It may be possible to test out certain parts but not all of this theory. *Mid-range theories* are narrower in scope and seek to deal with a particular aspect of the world. They are more likely to be testable and usable. Many nursing theories, for example that designed by Peplau, fall into this category. *Practice theories* focus on particular events, for example the formation of pressure sores or pain relief, and should therefore be testable and usable (Walker and Avant 1988).

Reading

> **Reading Suggestion 2.1**
>
> 1. Example of a grand theory: Leininger, M. (1978) *Transcultural nursing: concepts, theories and practices*. John Wiley, New York.
> 2. Example of a mid-range theory: Peplau, H. (1952) *Interpersonal relations in nursing*. G.P. Putnam, New York.
> 3. Example of a practice theory: Norton, D. (1975) *An investigation of geriatric problems in hospital*. Churchill Livingstone, Edinburgh.

Within all these categories the purpose of theory (Fawcett 1989) is to

either
• describe/classify/inform about events or situations;
or
• explain events or situations;
or
• predict outcomes.

APPLYING THEORY IN PRACTICE

Exercise 2.2 How do you use theory?

Choose an everyday event in your practice and try to identify how you use theory to inform your practice.

Exercises

Example 1

Mrs Jones underwent a mastectomy yesterday. Which theories would you draw on in order to provide care in the first 24 hours?

Your answer might include:

Discipline	Theory about
Physiology	Pain and the most effective way to provide pain relief. Wound care to prevent infection and promote healing. Respiration and the effects of anaesthetic. The circulation of the blood and the prevention of stasis.
Psychology	Loss and altered body image.
Nursing	The aims of nursing Mrs Jones, how these aims can be achieved by integrating theories from other disciplines into nursing care.

Theory can be used to *describe* the immediate post-operative phase. For example the condition of the wound, blood pressure and the degree of pain experienced by Mrs Jones. It may be used to *explain* to her and her husband how the wound will heal, the nature and importance of post-operative exercises and the fitting of a prosthesis. It may be used to *predict* outcomes, for example in terms of adaptation to altered body image, possible wound or chest infections. It will therefore enable the nurse to take action to prevent post-operative problems.

Example 2

Mr Smith is elderly and lives alone in a property which he cannot afford to maintain. He tends to drink heavily. Which theories would you draw on if you went to visit him at home?

Your answer might include:

Discipline	Theory about
Psychology	Interpersonal interaction. Assessing mental health status and cognitive abilities. Factors such as bereavement, and loneliness which may be present. Ageing.

Sociology   Poverty and its effects.
                  Social networks.
Physiology   Effects of alcohol on body systems.
                  Effects of ageing.
Nursing   Individualized and holistic approaches to assessing, planning, implementing and evaluating the care which Mr Smith requires.

Theory may be used to *describe* the situation in which Mr Smith lives, as a basis for assessment and identification of his particular difficulties. It may be used to *explain* to Mr Smith why certain health problems have arisen. It can also be used to advocate on his behalf in order to help him improve his circumstances. Finally theory can be used to *predict* outcomes, for example in relation to alcohol abuse or the increased effects of old age, so that the nurse can plan ahead.

DEVELOPING THEORY

A theory represents the thinking of an individual who is attempting to provide an explanation of something or a new interpretation of it. The theorist has to have imagination in order to see new possibilities, relationships or opportunities especially in matters which may have been taken for granted for years. The theorist also needs creativity to investigate and establish these possibilities, relationships and opportunities. Theory development is therefore a creative process. The same concepts may be used in different theories but linked in different ways and new theory should contribute in some way to our understanding of the world around us.

In considering this creative element, it can be helpful to look not only at the theory itself but also at the factors which may have influenced the theorist's thinking, creativity, choice of method used to develop the theory and the nature of the theory itself. In this context we might consider issues such as the professional background of the theorist, including training and experience. For example, Leininger trained as a nurse and anthropologist. Her theory of transcultural nursing reflects a blend of the two disciplines. Alternatively we could identify individuals who have influenced the theorist. For example Roy was taught by Dorothy Johnson who had herself designed a systems-based theory of nursing. Johnson challenged Roy to develop her own theory (Blue *et al.* 1989) based on research. The influence of systems-based theory can be clearly seen in Roy's work. The society and period in which the theory was developed is an additional factor for consideration. For example in Roger's theory the environment for nursing extends into all areas: home, school work, leisure both on earth and in outer space (Daily *et al.* 1989). Whilst this may at first sound preposterous it is important to remember that Rogers developed her theory during the 1960s when the idea of travelling to and living on other planets seemed an imminent possibility.

EVALUATING THEORY

Reading

> **Reading Suggestion 2.2**
>
> The skills of evaluating research are described by Avis, 1994. Avis, M. (1994) Reading research critically, 1. *Journal of Clinical Nursing* 3, 227–234; Avis, M. (1994) Reading research critically 2. An introduction to appraisal: assessing the evidence. *Journal of Clinical Nursing* 3, 271–277.

Practitioners have the responsibility of deciding for themselves whether they accept a theory and wish to use it in their practice or not. Each practitioner needs to examine specific theories critically to determine whether they are applicable in his/her professional field. In looking at any theory there are a number of questions we can ask which will help us decide whether or not it will be helpful to us. This critical appraisal involves examining the strengths and weaknesses of the theory and making judgements about both the theory itself and its usefulness. In may ways the skills involved are similar to evaluating a piece of research. It is important to stress that being critical is not the same as being destructive. A true critical appraisal should aim to give a balanced, informed view of the theory, not tear it apart. The questions in Exercise 2.3 are intended to help you with the task of critical appraisal. You might like to try this exercise on your own or in a small group. The questions may be photocopied.

Exercises

> **Exercise 2.3 Evaluating theory**
>
> Choose *one* theory with which you feel familiar and which you use. Try to answer the following questions in relation to the theory. Examples might include nursing theories such as those of Orem or Peplau. Alternatively you could choose a theory from another field such as physiology or psychology if you regularly use these within your sphere of practice.
>
> 1. What is the background of the theorist?
> 2. Which concepts are used in the theory?
> 3. What methods were used to develop the theory?
> 4. How clear is the theory?
> 5. What does the theory say?
> 6. What type of theory is it?
> 7. Can the theory be used?
> 8. Is the theory relevant to the clinical area in which I work?
> 9. Is the theory important?
> 10. How feasible would it be to implement the theory? For example, would it fit in with the existing situation or would this have to be changed to accommodate the theory? What would be the cost of such changes both in financial and other terms?
> 11. Is there a need for a trial first?
> 12. Is the theory congruent with patients' expectations?
> 13. Is the practitioner covered by law to apply this theory?
> 14. Has the theory been critically examined by others in the same field?

Evaluating Peplau's theory of psychodynamic nursing

1.   What is the background of the theorist?

An American nurse who qualified in 1931, Peplau had considerable experience in mental health. Her clinical experience brought her into contact with some of the foremost psychiatrists of the day. Major influences included Sullivan, Fromm and Maslow. She began publishing her ideas in the early 1950s. In addition to developing her theory, she influenced psychiatric nursing in many ways, for example she launched the first postgraduate course in this field thus establishing psychiatric nursing as a speciality at a time when the clinical nurse specialist and advanced practice roles in most other branches of nursing were only beginning to emerge (Carey *et al.* 1989).

2.   Which concepts are used in the theory?

(a)   The nurse–patient relationship. This has four phases: orientation, identification, exploitation and resolution. In the orientation phase the nurse and patient meet as strangers. They work collaboratively to clarify the patient's problem. In the identification phase the patient responds to those who can meet his/her needs. This response can be passive, dependent on the nurse; participatory and interdependent with the nurse; autonomous and independent of the nurse. In the exploitation phase the patient starts to become more independent but still needs some support. In resolution the patient's needs have been met and the nurse–patient relationship should be brought to a close (Peplau 1952, Carey *et al.* 1989).

(b)   Psychodynamic nursing. This concept is about the interpersonal processes between the nurse and the patient. Peplau regarded illness as a potential learning experience for both parties through which both can grow and develop. The nurse had to become a mature person in order to be of help to patients. Psychodynamic nursing is therefore the central concept in the theory underpinning all the others (Peplau 1952, Carey *et al.* 1989).

(c)   Nursing roles. Peplau identifies six nursing roles: stranger, resource, teacher, leader, counsellor and surrogate. With the exception of stranger, these roles are not used in any particular order. The nurse and patient meet as strangers. Each should be afforded the courtesy due to strangers. This meeting is the basis for the nurse–patient relationship and psychodynamic nursing. The nurse can adopt the role of resource person by providing useful information and acting as a source of referral. If necessary the nurse can teach the patient new knowledge and skills to facilitate management of the illness or a return to normal life. The nurse acts as a leader in promoting the independence of the patient enabling him/her to make decisions. The role of counsellor enables the patient to become more aware of what is happening as a result of illness and to develop appropriate coping strategies. In the surrogate role the nurse acts as a significant other to help the patient deal with specific problems (Simpson 1991).

3. *What methods were used to develop the theory?*

Peplau drew on a number of established theories available at the time, for example those of Maslow and Sullivan. She synthesized these in the development of her own theory. Further refinement came through clinical work and teaching (Carey *et al.* 1989).

4. *How clear is the theory?*

The theory is clearly presented and easily understood. Terminology is clear and consistent.

5. *What does the theory say?*

The theory states that the nurse–patient relationship is of central importance for both parties. The way in which the two interact has significant implications for the patient's progress. The nurse can benefit the patient by adopting certain roles which require a wide repertoire of skills. If the nurse is to be able to establish therapeutic relationships with patients, s/he must develop and grow as a person. Nursing can therefore be described as 'a maturing force that aims to promote forward movement of personality in the direction of creative, constructive, productive, personal and community living' (Peplau 1952).

6. *What type of theory is it?*

This is a mid-range theory (Fawcett 1995) which can be tested in practice.

7. *Can the theory be used?*

The theory has been used by a number of practitioners both within and outside the mental health field. Hall, a District Nurse, applied the theory in caring for a man with AIDS and found that

> Peplau's framework for care gave me the guidance and direction I needed to obtain a positive outcome in this situation. Like Peplau, I believe that individuals are capable of achieving new learning and making positive changes . . . but at the beginning of the case I wondered whether I would actually achieve anything with my client. (Hall 1994)

In a North American study, Jewell and Sullivan (1996) successfully applied Peplau's theory with health education groups. Morrison *et al.* (1996), another American team, used the theory to examine the work roles of staff nurses in mental health settings. Their examples seem to confirm Fawcett's (1995) argument that Peplau's theory is in the mid-range category and is therefore usable.

8.   Is the theory relevant to the clinical area in which I work?

This is a question which only individual practitioners can answer. Peplau's theory stresses the importance of the nurse–patient relationship. If that relationship is central to nursing practice, then Peplau's ideas are relevant to all clinical areas. There may, however, be degrees of relevance. The phases of the relationship and the possible roles which the nurse can adopt take time to develop. In some instances, these could take weeks or even months. In settings with a high patient turnover, such as day surgery, nurse–patient relationships can be severely curtailed (Simpson 1991). Consequently practitioners have to decide the extent to which they can apply Peplau's theory based on the amount of time available for the development of relationships.

Discussion

> **Discussion Topic 2.3**
>
> What do you see as the strengths and weaknesses of Peplau's theory in relation to your field of practice?

9.   Is the theory important?

The theory is important, first of all, because it is an early attempt to devise a theory of nursing. Also, despite its age, it seems to reflect the realities of nursing practice in a variety of different settings. However, the practitioner must also ask 'is it important for the area in which I work and if so, in what way?'

10.   How feasible would it be to implement the theory? Would it fit in with the existing situation or would this have to be changed to accommodate the theory? What would be the cost of such changes both in financial and other terms?

Implementing this theory requires some degree of nursing skill largely because Peplau does not provide a clear guide to assessment. This is partly because her work pre-dates the introduction of the nursing process. More importantly, for the nurse to meet the patient with a prepared checklist tips the balance between them. They do not meet as strangers, in equality, and without preconceived ideas about one another.

Holt (1988) has demonstrated application of the orientation stage of the theory, in the care of a patient with acute myocardial infarction. His assessment was carried out using a blank sheet of paper 'but, because of a lack of familiarity with non-structured assessment, the writer prepared a list of possible questions to guide the conversation if it appeared to flag or go off at a tangent'. Holt also comments on the difficulty in recording all that is said in an assessment of this type. Instead he recorded 'points mutually agreed to be significant' (Holt 1988).

Hall (1994) also had some difficulty with the idea of unstructured assessment and, in addition, was obliged to use the nursing documentation approved by her employers. She therefore combined Peplau's theory with the assessment tool based on Roper, Logan and Tierney's (1990) Activities of Living. Unstructured assessment can therefore be said to raise issues about nursing documentation. Existing paperwork is probably unsuitable for this type of assessment. Nursing teams would therefore have to consider how they would record unstructured assessments in order to ensure that the information obtained was accessible to all staff. Teams would also have to ensure that their managers were familiar with and supported the use of, such an approach to assessment.

An additional consideration is the emphasis which Peplau places on the nurse–patient relationship which can create a considerable burden for the nurse and may even involve risks. In order to act as a therapeutic agent the nurse has to have a wide range of skills and knowledge. The willingness to be open with the patient, learn from the patient, and adopt roles such as counsellor, can create immense stress. Consequently the nurse needs a support system (Simpson 1991) which is both non-judgmental and non-punitive and which will allow each practitioner to achieve the necessary personal growth.

In considering these issues it is evident that the introduction of Peplau's theory would require a staff education programme. The aims of this programme would be to ensure that everyone understood the theory, to promote discussion about its application and to ensure agreement about how it should be implemented. In addition staff would require some practice in applying the theory with their patients. Support systems would have to be developed. Management education and support would also be essential because of the changes in working practice and the documentation of nursing care. Financial costs are inherent in all of these issues.

11.   Is there a need for a trial first?

In view of the preparatory work needed to introduce the theory, a trial period is probably advisable.

12.   Is the theory congruent with patients' expectations?

What is it that your patients want when they come to you for nursing care? The simplest answer is to ask them. Buehler (1992) asked a local Crow Indian population what doctors and nurses needed to know in order to provide care. Results showed how much the Indians valued the use of indigenous healers and traditional healing practices and the need for professionals to respect these. Seeking the views of patients is a burgeoning industry in health care. You may find it helpful to look at what your organization is doing about this and the results obtained in trying to decide whether Peplau's theory will suit your clients.

13. Is the practitioner covered by law to enact this theory?

Yes. This theory conforms to the legal requirements for nursing practice. It is also in line with professional requirements as set out in the Scope of Professional Practice (UKCC 1992).

14. Has the theory been critically examined by others in the same field?

Simpson (1991) critically examined Peplau's theory using five care studies which included a child, an elderly person and patients with mental health problems. His approach demonstrates that the phases of the nurse–patient relationship are relevant in getting to know a patient and enable the nurse to implement the nursing process. However, issues such as the time required to develop the nurse–patient relationship, nursing documentation and staff support need to be taken into consideration. The role of counsellor is particularly important in Peplau's theory but 'not everyone who gives nursing care feels comfortable counselling, where it is the patient who has control in the situation. The only control the nurse exercises is in directing the discussion by the questions she asks. Less experienced carers may shift control in their own favour by resorting to advising' (Simpson 1991).

Morrison *et al.* (1996) also identified the importance of the counselling role. They recorded 62 nurse–patient interactions between staff nurses in mental health settings and patients. Adults, children and adolescents were included in the sample. Results showed that counsellor was the role most often adopted by the nurses. Overlap between other roles, such as resource and teacher, was also apparent.

SUMMARY

The aim of this chapter has been to introduce you to the concept of theory and the questions you might ask about any theory regardless of whether it arises from within nursing or elsewhere. It may seem strange to begin this book by asking you to evaluate a theory but it is hoped that this will help you to read critically as you encounter the different types of theory presented in this book. I hope that you will return to this exercise again as you read the book and that it will be helpful to you in developing a questioning approach to your practice.

This chapter has also raised the question of how much we use theory as an integral part of our daily practice. Most of the time we do not think of our work as being theoretically based but the truth is that we cannot nurse in any other way. If we don't know and use theory from nursing and from other disciplines then we are simply carrying out a series of tasks based on ignorance. I hope that the following chapters will help you reappraise the position of theory in your practice.

REFERENCES

Blue, C., Brubaker, K., Fine, J., Kirsch, M., Papazian, K. and Riester, C. (1989) *Sister Callista Roy: Adaptation model. In:* Marriner-Twomey, A. (ed.) (1989) *Nursing theorists and their work*, 2nd edn, CV Mosby, St Louis.

Buehler, J. (1992) Traditional Crow Indian health beliefs and practices. *Journal of Holistic Nursing* 10 (1), 18–33.

Carey, E., Noll, J., Rasmussen, L., Searcy, B. and Stark, N. (1989) *Hildegard E. Peplau. Psychodynamic nursing. In:* Marriner-Twomey, A. (ed.) *Nursing theorists and their work*, 2nd edn, CV Mosby, St Louis.

Chinn, P. and Kramer, M. (1991) *Theory and nursing*, 3rd edn, Mosby Year Book, St Louis.

Chinn, P. and Kramer, M. (1995) *Theory and nursing*, 4th edn, Mosby Year Book, St Louis.

Clifford, C. (1995) Caring: fitting the concept into nursing practice. *Journal of Clinical Nursing* 4, 37–41.

Daily, J., Maupin, J., Satterly, M., Schnell, D. and Wallace, T. (1989) *Martha E. Rogers. Unitary beings. In:* Marriner-Twomey, A. (ed.), *Nursing theorists and their work*, 2nd edn, CV Mosby, St Louis.

Dickoff, J. and James, P. (1968) A theory of theories: a position paper, *Nursing Research* 17 (3), 197–203.

Fawcett, J. (1989) *Analysis and evaluation of conceptual models of nursing*, 2nd edn, F.A. Davis, Philadelphia.

Fawcett, J. (1995) *Analysis and evaluation of conceptual models of nursing*, 3rd edn, F.A. Davis, Philadelphia.

Fawcett, J. and Downs, F. (1992) *The relationship of theory and research*, 2nd edn, F.A. Davis, Philadelphia.

Hall, K. (1994) Peplau's model of nursing: caring for a man with AIDS. *British Journal of Nursing* 13 (8), 418–422.

Holt, T. (1988) *Care plan for a man following a myocardial infarction, using Peplau's developmental model. In*: Chalmers, H. (1988) (ed.) *Choosing a model. Caring for patients with cardiovascular and respiratory problems*, Edward Arnold, London.

Jewell, J. and Sullivan, E. (1996) Application of nursing theories in health education. *Journal of the American Psychiatric Nurses Association* 2 (3), 79–85.

Kech, J. (1989) *Terminology of theory development. In:* Marriner-Twomey, A. (ed.), *Nursing theorists and their work*, 2nd edn, CV Mosby, St Louis.

Morrison, E., Shealy, A., Kowalski, C., LaMont, J. and Range, B. (1996) Work roles of staff nurses in psychiatric settings. *Nursing Science Quarterly* 9 (1), 17–21.

Peplau, H. (1952) *Interpersonal relations in nursing*, G.P. Putnam, New York.

Roper, N., Logan, W. and Tierney, A. (1990) *The elements of nursing*, 3rd edn, Churchill Livingstone, Edinburgh.

Schrodinger, E. (1951) *Science and Humanisim.* Cambridge University Press, Cambridge. *Quoted in* Zukav, G. (1991) *The dancing Wu Li Masters*, 2nd edn, Rider, London.

Simpson, H. (1991) *Peplau's model in action*, Macmillan, Basingstoke.

United Kingdom Central Council for Nursing Midwifery and Health Visiting (1992) *The scope of professional practice*, UKCC, London.

Walker, L. and Avant, K. (1988) *Strategies for theory construction in nursing*, 2nd edn, Appleton Lange, Norwalk, Connecticut.

Nursing and theory | 3

WHAT IS NURSING?

In the previous chapter we explored the concept of theory in a broad way which could apply to any theory from any discipline. In this chapter we will look in more detail at theory in nursing, why we need it and some of the ideas which have shaped current professional thought. This will involve learning some new terminology which will be helpful in reading about specific theories. In addition this chapter will examine the assumption that there is a division between the theory and the practice of nursing. In order to address these issues, it is necessary to consider what nursing is and what it does, which means looking beyond the definitions we were given as students to a deeper and more comprehensive picture.

Each profession has to identify those aspects of the world with which it will concern itself and the unique manner in which it will do so (McGee 1993). Failure to do this means a lack of agreement on the proper work of the profession and, consequently, confusion. The proverbial wheel has to be constantly re-invented. Agreement on what the profession will do, its functions and remit, allows practitioners to get on with the task in hand and must be sufficiently flexible to cover a variety of settings (Chalmers 1982). It will also form the basis for professional knowledge. The global view of the profession as a whole, the concepts, ideas, theories etc. of which it is composed is sometimes called a metaparadigm. There are several different explanations of the nursing metaparadigm available to us. Two of them are considered here.

Reading Suggestion 3.1

Read Chalmers, A. (1982) *What is this thing called science?* 2nd edn, Open University Press, Buckingham. Chapter 8, Theories and structures. Critically examine the ideas it presents in relation to nursing.

Reading

CARPER'S EXPLANATION OF NURSING

According to Carper (1978) nursing has four dimensions: *empirical, ethical, personal and aesthetic*. In her original paper these are only briefly set out

Empirical dimension	Ethical dimension
Describing	Valuing
Explaining	Clarifying
Predicting	Advocating
Personal dimension	Aesthetic dimension
Being open	Engaging
Reflecting	Interpreting
Realizing the	Creating
genuine self	

Fig. 3.1 Carper's explanation of nursing. Based on Carper (1978), Chinn and Kramer (1991, 1995).

but later writers, particularly Chinn and Kramer (1995) have developed her ideas further.

In the dimension of empirical knowledge, nursing draws on areas of science such as physiology, microbiology and pharmacology. In these fields knowledge arises from what can be observed, measured and tested. At the most elementary level empirical knowledge describes situations; at the next it attempts to explain and at the most sophisticated, to predict (Chinn and Kramer 1995) (Figure 3.1).

In the ethical dimension, nursing is concerned with making judgments about what ought/ought not to be done, what is acceptable behaviour in certain circumstances. At the elementary level ethical knowledge is about identifying values. Those of the patients, the nurses, the profession and the employers are all included here. Clarifying comes next. This involves examining the reasons behind particular values and how values interrelate. At its most advanced level, the ethical dimension of nursing enables the nurse to act as advocate (Chinn and Kramer 1995) (Figure 3.1).

The personal dimension refers to the personal growth and development of each nurse. It acknowledges that the nurse is a human being with qualities which may affect therapeutic interactions with patients. Ideally such qualities should be positive, enabling the individual nurse to function in unique ways. Negative qualities need to be examined and managed in a way which minimizes their effect on the nurse–patient relationship. The most elementary level of the personal dimension of nursing is that of being open to other people, to new ideas and experiences. The ability to reflect on these factors follows on from this and is instrumental in enabling the nurse to develop insight into other views of the world, including those of patients. At the third stage is self-awareness, which is a 'process of express-ing through personality, behaviour, words and deeds the genuine, real whole self that is consistent with what is experienced in the inner life' (Chinn and Kramer 1991) (Figure 3.1).

In the aesthetic dimension there is integration of the empirical, ethical and personal dimensions to enable the nurse to act as a therapeutic agent and create new possibilities for the patient. Initially this means getting involved in the patient's situation, meeting the patient in an open, genuine manner. The nurse is then able to interpret what is happening in the situation; identifying, explaining and predicting problems. Finally, at the most sophisticated level, the nurse is creative: able to identify and develop a range of possible solutions to the situation and select that which is most appropriate.

This explanation was developed at a time when there was considerable emphasis on nursing as a science, possibly to the detriment of other aspects of the nurse's role. Carper's ideas help to redress the imbalance between the scientific and artistic domains of practice. In addition, she acknowledges that nurses are individual human beings rather than the pairs of hands described by researchers such as Menzies (1970). An additional strength of Carper's explanation is that it helps us analyse a situation in terms of what the nurse is doing even in small, daily tasks like giving out medicines.

Exercise 3.1 Application of Carper's explanation of nursing

One of the questions we should ask about Carper's ideas is whether they are still applicable to nursing today. In order to test this out (Fig. 3.2), select one nursing situation and explore how far Carper's ideas can be applied.

Exercises

However, Carper herself made no attempt to link the four dimensions with what nurses actually do and consequently applying these ideas is difficult, as you may have found (Fig. 3.2). Despite the integrating nature of

Empirical dimension

Describing: the nurse can identify the medication and can describe its function.

Explaining: the nurse teaches the patient about taking his medication, why it should be taken at a particular time, the importance of completing the course, common side effects, etc.

Predicting: the nurse is able to recognize whether the patient is able to comply with instructions regarding his medication, to anticipate and try to minimize any risks involved.

Personal dimension

Being open: the nurse is able to be open and non-judgmental about the situation and is also aware of personal strengths and weaknesses in dealing with this sort of matter.

Reflecting: the nurse reflects on the patient's actions and opinions and integrates these with past experiences.

Realizing: the nurse is able to act in a genuine manner, to be a resource for the patient.

Ethical dimension

Valuing: the nurse identifies the differing values of the personnel involved in the situation: the patient, nursing staff, medical staff, relatives (possibly) and local policy. For example the patient may be afraid of receiving medication by injection whereas the doctor may feel that this is the best route for administration

Clarifying: the nurse clarifies the different value systems of those involved. For example the patient may have had frightening experiences in the past or may come from a culture in which certain routes of administration are considered superior to others.

Advocating: the nurse enables the patient to make his views heard.

Aesthetic dimension

Engaging: the nurse gets involved in the situation, without judging anyone.

Interpreting: the nurse is able to hone in on what is important in the situation, possibly without even realizing that this is happening.

Creativity: the nurse is able to be a therapeutic agent, creating and using appropriate strategies to resolve the situation.

Fig. 3.2 Application of Carper's explanation of nursing.

aesthetics, the division of nursing knowledge into compartments (Sweeney 1994) does not encourage the nurse to use knowledge or skills which might overlap or be transferred between dimensions. Therefore an holistic approach to patient care may be lost.

It could also be argued that nursing has developed considerably as a profession since 1978. For example, the amount of legislation of relevance to nursing practice has increased dramatically and might even be enough to form a separate dimension. There is now a far greater emphasis on health, health promotion and health education, none of which feature in Carper's work. Consequently her ideas could be said to be somewhat dated. Metaparadigms such as these will continue only so long as there is a large enough consensus to support them. Inevitably, new developments, new knowledge presents a challenge to an accepted explanation which may be able to incorporate these new ideas. If it cannot do so, then rival, potential explanations will emerge and in time a new one will predominate, replacing the old (Chalmers 1982).

Discussion

> **Discussion Topic 3.1**
>
> What elements do you think should be included in Carper's explanation and why?

FAWCETT'S EXPLANATION OF NURSING

According to Fawcett (1995) nursing also has four dimensions (Fig. 3.3). The *person* is the recipient of nursing activity and may thus be an individual, a family or a group. The *environment* is the setting in which the person lives and therefore incorporates both home, work and other places, as well as the people to whom the person is emotionally close. The environment includes the settings in which nursing activities take place. *Health* is the person's state of being; what is normal for him/her. It is more than the absence of illness. Finally, *nursing* refers to the activities of a qualified professional nurse in assessing, planing, implementing and evaluating nursing services for the person.

Each dimension can be examined individually as shown in later chapters of this book but Fawcett (1995) emphasizes that they are each interrelated. Health or the lack of it are integral parts of the person's life. Factors within

Person	Health
Environment	Nursing

Fig. 3.3 Fawcett's explanation of nursing (1995).

Table 3.1 Categories of nursing theories. The commonest categories are listed here. For others please see Fawcett (1995)

1.	Developmental	Emphasize the processes of growth, development, and maturation. Focus on change, seeing the person over time.
		Example: Roper, Logan and Tierney.
2.	Systems	See the person as made up of systems. These systems are open, in constant interaction with each other and the environment. Systems are subject to stresses and strains but strive towards equilibrium.
		Example: Roy
3.	Interactions	Are concerned with interpersonal relationships and how people communicate with one another.
		Example: Peplau.

the person and the environment will affect the individual's experience of health. The person cannot be separated from his/her environment and there is interaction between the two. Nursing is concerned with health and with facilitating the achievement of health within both the person and the environment.

This explanation dominates current writing and thinking about nursing. Nursing theories are structured and expressed in relation to these four elements, acceptance of which allows nurses to develop their own approaches to practice creatively. Thus whilst we have many different types of nursing theory, Fawcett's explanation is sufficiently broad to accommodate them. Consequently, it is possible to have many different, and even conflicting, models of nursing based on this single explanation (Table 3.1).

Discussion Topic 3.2

Compare and contrast *two* theories of nursing in terms of what each says about nursing. Do you agree or disagree? Give reasons.

Discussion

It can be difficult to take a step back and look critically at Fawcett's ideas because they underpin so much of our professional thinking, whether or not we are aware of this. It could be argued that, unlike Carper, this modern explanation of nursing tries to take an holistic approach by showing the interrelatedness of the four dimensions. In doing so it appears to be more comprehensive and perhaps more neutral than Carper's work in that the four dimensions are open to interpretation by individual nurses in a wide variety of settings.

However, if Fawcett's overall explanation of nursing is truly neutral then it should function internationally and not reflect 'particular national, cultural, or ethnic beliefs and values' (Fawcett 1995). It must be acknowledged that this is not the case and this in itself may account for some of the difficulties nurses experience in applying theory to practice. The concepts of person, environment, health and nursing appear to be neutral but it is possible that they are still rooted in particular cultures and may therefore not be applicable on a truly international basis. We should not therefore assume that this metaparadigm is fixed and unchangeable.

ADVANTAGES OF A GLOBAL EXPLANATION OF NURSING

This discussion about the nature of nursing may seem rather abstract and far removed from the real world of nursing practice. Does it really matter whether there is an agreed explanation of what nursing is? Some might argue that they are quite able to get on and nurse patients without 'all this theory'. What then are Carper and Fawcett giving us as nurses?

To begin with they are enabling us to identify those activities which are solely the domain of the nurse as opposed to any other professional/lay group. It is possible that neither Carper or Fawcett have produced an explanation which serves the whole of nursing. Professionally speaking we may still be at the stage of re-inventing the wheel. Alternatively we could look on Carper and Fawcett as challenging an existing definition of our work. We may disagree with everything presented here, but at least we have a starting point for determining what we think nursing is. This is essential if we are to promote nursing within the organizations in which we work. In the purchaser–provider economy of the health service we need to be proactive not only in deciding what we can realistically provide by way of services but in convincing purchasers of the reasons why they should employ nurses in preference to less qualified staff.

Both Carper's and Fawcett's ideas provide the basis for a language in which nurses can talk about nursing. We all know the language of other health care professions, particularly medicine. For example we understand what is meant by congestive cardiac failure, cerebrovascular accident and cholecystectomy. Medical language provides a common currency for communication between doctors and between doctors and other professionals, both within the immediate health care setting and in the wider arena. In contrast the language of nursing is far less well developed. Carper and Fawcett's contributions therefore represent an important step in enabling the profession to discuss nursing in its own terms.

Reading

> **Reading Suggestion 3.2**
>
> Look up references to the North American Nursing Diagnosis Association (NANDA). In what ways could this type of work help develop a language for nursing?

Allied to these concepts of professional language and discussion is that of education. A metaparadigm provides a coherent framework for education (Draper 1990) without which it is almost impossible to explain what we do. Without it one is drawn into listing tasks which by themselves have no meaning, no goal and might be performed by anybody (Cook 1991).

Carper and Fawcett's ideas therefore raise nursing above this, by identifying a body of theoretical knowledge which underpins and directs nursing actions.

Finally their work provides a basis for nurses to generate and test out new theories about nursing practice. Every nurse has a responsibility towards the development of practice though individuals' degree of involvement in this may vary. However there is no logical reason why any nurse cannot develop his/her own theory about some aspect of practice. Most nurses have some thoughts about this, but unfortunately most carry their ideas in their heads without ever attempting to make them explicit (Fawcett 1989, McGee 1993) because they are misled into thinking that only published theories will be taken seriously. Consequently nurses lack confidence in developing their own ideas and may even think that they have no role to play in professional discourse. The result is a perception of theoretical ideas as being outside practice, separate and even irrelevant to it.

THE SEPARATION OF THEORY AND PRACTICE IN NURSING

There are of course other reasons for this perceived gap between theory and practice and there is a considerable amount of literature on this topic which can be summarized in terms of:

- divisions among nurses;
- divisions between curricula;
- divisions between theory and nurses.

Divisions among nurses

'Nurses never stick together!' It is a common enough complaint especially when nurses feel threatened and under pressure. To some extent the complaint is justified because some groups within nursing do seem to distance themselves from others. The problem lies in establishing who is distancing themselves, from whom and why. To answer some of these questions it is necessary to look back over the last fifteen years.

Miller (1985) argues that the two camps are the practitioners and the educational theorists (Table 3.2). The two differ in terms of education, employment, perceptions of patients and perceptions of nursing. The divisions between the two camps are sustained by many factors. Language is perhaps the greatest of them all. Miller cites a letter in the *Nursing Times* in which the writer complains about a particular model saying:

> I suspect many of us cannot understand it . . . I am skeptical whether consideration of the supply of sustenal imperatives to the eliminative subsystem will do much to alert the nurse of a particular patient's need for brown bread for breakfast.

Added to this is the divergence between the ideal as perceived by the educationalists and the reality as experienced by the practitioners. The two

Table 3.2 Divisions between practitioners and educational theorists

	Practitioner	Educational theorist
Background & education	Trained nurse working in a massive bureaucracy	Trained professional working in educational establishment
Employment situation	One of a group of nurses caring for a group of patients	One nurse teaching about hypothetical patients
Perception of nursing	Nursing is what it is	Focus on what it ought to be
	Mainly about doing	Mainly about knowing
	Value experience and tradition	Value knowledge based on research
Nursing knowledge	Passed on by oral tradition and example	Passed on through teaching and writing
Perceptions	Fragmented view; passive recipients of care all treated alike	Overly comprehensive view; emphasize individuality, health and active participation in care

(Adapted from Miller 1985)

groups ask different questions about nursing. For example, practitioners tend to question methods and draw on past experience. They rarely question their underlying knowledge base, whereas educational theorists tend to do just that and then point out how little of nursing actually arises from sound scientific knowledge.

Miller's analysis offers us a straightforward division between those who generate theory and those who do the 'real work' of nursing. In contrast, White's (1985) analysis shows three camps whose divisions are centred on the organization of the nursing service. The generalists see nursing primarily as a practical job. They tend to accept the hierarchical structure within nursing; see no need for any qualifications beyond initial training and are happy to work under the supervision of managers. The generalist's sense of status is derived from his/her position in the hierarchy.

The specialists have usually undertaken additional training; value status based on education; tend to challenge the status quo and prefer to work without supervision. The managers work predominantly outside the nursing setting and consequently tend to adopt the norms of their bureaucratic colleagues. They have little or no formal training for their roles and have a history of trying to control other nurses, especially the specialists. Consequently there is conflict between the managers and the specialists.

Both Miller and White argue that divisions among nurses are based on widely differing educational backgrounds and attitudes to nursing work. These differences affect the ways in which members of the two camps interact. Specialists challenge the managers who react by trying to control them. Educational theorists and practitioners do not even share a common language. It is but a small step from there for members of each camp to accuse those of the other of not living in the real world; of being impractical and of talking nonsense.

Nowhere are the divisions between nurses more apparent at the moment than in the separation of nurse teachers from other nurses. To some extent teachers have always separated themselves from those they taught in the belief that familiarity would undermine their ability to function and, in particular, give correction to students. Such separation is also part of the system by which education can reinforce patterns of social class, sexual identities and language. However, what in the past could be termed social distance, is now developing into a physical separation between those who teach and those who practice nursing (Ferguson and Jinks 1994). As colleges of nursing move into higher education the nurse teacher will become more isolated from clinical nursing colleagues. The travelling and sheer effort required to find time to visit clinical areas may compound the problem. Consequently there is the possibility that, like the managers in White's analysis, nurse teachers begin to take on the norms of other staff groups such as those within the university.

Attempts to overcome the separation

In the past there have been several attempts to overcome this separation of teachers and practitioners, most notably through:

(a) *Registered Clinical Nurse Teachers (RCNT)* who were introduced in the 1950s and were intended to be practice-based, working with the students, performing hands-on care. They received less training than the nurse tutors, experienced low status and had no career prospects unless they went on to undertake a nurse tutor course or returned to clinical practice full time (Lathlean 1995). Research conducted by the Royal College of Nursing led to recommendations by the College that there should be only one grade of nurse teacher and that this grade should be able to teach both in the classroom and in the clinical setting (RCN 1983, Crotty and Butterworth 1992). Since then there has been a national trend to abandon the RCNT grade although according to Clifford (1993) it is still possible to register as a clinical teacher by obtaining a Diploma in Nursing and completing a City and Guilds course.

(b) *Tutor liaison*, in which a tutor is assigned to a specific clinical area. This role can be used by itself or in conjunction with other activities such as regular meetings between the tutor and the clinical staff; joint teaching sessions by the tutor and clinical staff (Khadim and Wafer 1993). It has the potential to be very successful but the concept of liaison must be made completely clear (Clifford 1993) or staff, students and tutors experience dissatisfaction.

(c) The introduction of the *lecturer-practitioner* – a senior nurse who 'is appointed by both a trust and a university or who has responsibilities to both a trust and a university' (Fairbrother and Ford 1996). The lecturer-practitioner has both a teaching and a practice role and must be credible in both fields. According to Lathlean (1992) these nurses do not see themselves as bridging the theory–practice gap but the joint nature of their responsibilities may enable them to do so by supporting staff at differing stages in their careers (Woodrow 1994). However the realities of dual responsibilities may create considerable stress particularly if the two sets of managers do not share the same view of the post (Dearmun 1993). The lecturer-practitioner can end up carrying a full workload in each setting with managers and colleagues having very little idea what the postholder does when not on their patch.

Limitations of these initiatives

The central weakness in all these initiatives is the implicit assumption that one person can change the world; that, by installing an individual who can function in both the educational and the practice settings, the gulf between the two will disappear. This places an enormous burden on the individual who, of course, carries the blame if the world remains unchanged. It may be that what is needed is complete organizational change to create a climate in which education and practice share a common organizational structure which encompasses all professionals. In the Rush unification model of practice, all staff, in all professions and whatever grade, practice, teach and are involved in research. The percentage of time devoted to each activity depends on the nature of their post (Cochran *et al.* 1989).

In the meantime, the current situation in nurse education within the UK requires some imaginative work on the part of nurse teachers and their practice based colleagues, if they are to keep the communication channels open and maintain a professional respect for one another. The nurse teacher is now required to have 'relevant and up to date experience' as well as 'relevant and up to date research based expertise' (UKCC 1994). The nurse based in the clinical areas depends on the tutor for mandatory professional updating as well as post-registration education (UKCC 1994). Both camps need each other. Managers in higher education and in service have a responsibility to encourage innovative working relationships between practitioners and tutors. There must be emphasis in such innovations on regular and sustained commitment by tutors in the practice areas with the aim of achieving practice and educational development. The emphasis in such commitment must be on active participation in care delivery rather than observation from the sidelines. Managers also have a responsibility to encourage staff to publish accounts of these innovations and contribute to professional debate in this field.

Divisions between curricula

How often have you heard people say things like 'What is taught in the school is different to what you learn on the wards' or 'Never mind what you were taught in school; this is how we do it here.' In this analysis the divisions are not between nurses; they are between different sets of professional priorities which underpin what is taught to student nurses.

The student nurse encounters two distinct curricula. The overt curriculum (Cook 1991) is that which is intended and planned by the teaching staff. It is aimed at facilitating the acquisition of the formal knowledge and skill required to gain entry to the register of nurses. In contrast the covert curriculum is 'those non-academic but educationally significant consequences of schooling that occur systematically but are not made explicit at any level' (Cook 1991). This covert curriculum is focused on socializing the nurse into the culture of the profession and the particular hospital or organization. It is a combination, therefore, of preparing the student to be a 'good nurse' who will be sure of a job and 'the way we do things around here'. It is the 'unstated teaching of norms, attitudes and values to individual students through a process of meeting with the expectations of the institution' (Cook 1991).

Discussion Topic 3.3

How would you describe the two types of curriculum in your practice setting? Have they changed since the introduction of Project 2000 and, if so, how?

Discussion

Thus the student is exposed to two different curricula with very different aims and content. Both are essential to the student's development and nobody can say that one is better than the other. However there is inevitably tension between them because one is geared 'towards promoting social order and conformity' whilst the other 'has as its explicit aim the liberation and self-realization of the individual's potential, a potentially socially disruptive objective' (Cook 1991).

The existence of these two curricula is not new. As a tutor in charge of pre-Project 2000 courses I was well aware of, and at times depended on the covert curriculum to address the issues involved in socializing new students into nursing. At the end of an introductory course, I knew I could rely on the ward sisters to inculcate, for example, the habit of punctuality in arriving on duty; coping with shift work and the delicate art of requesting off duty. Similarly, having trained in the same system, I knew all the tricks that students might get up to because I had used most of them myself.

What has brought the covert curriculum to the fore is the radical change in formal nurse education. The overt curriculum of Project 2000 is very different to what has gone before and this has created change in the covert curriculum. The problem is that neither teachers nor clinical nurses can say with confidence any longer that they know what the covert curriculum is. They can no longer assume that the student will acquire all the information needed in order to cope with the realities of working as a nurse.

Nurse teachers and clinical nurses have a joint responsibility to acknowledge openly the existence of both curricula and incorporate them in a joint effort to prepare students realistically for professional nursing practice (Cook 1991). This will mean having to demolish well established boundaries in terms of the knowledge base in each curriculum. The overt curriculum has emphasized factual knowledge (Dale 1994) and abstract goals such as self-directed learning (Ferguson and Jinks 1994). The covert curriculum has concentrated on the development of practical knowledge (Dale 1994) and safe, competent practitioners (Ferguson and Jinks 1994). For the student to truly benefit, both parties will have to learn something of each other's knowledge base and incorporate it into their own.

Divisions between theory and nurses

Nursing theory has an image problem which is largely of its own making. It has alienated nurses through its use of unfamiliar and difficult language. It relies on theories derived from other disciplines which it does not always use correctly and it has failed to reflect the realities of the nursing world in a way which is meaningful to the majority of nurses (Draper 1990, Tolley 1995). In this analysis the division is between the way in which theory is expressed and nursing as it is experienced by those in practice.

This is largely attributed to the import, from North America, of theories which are perceived as coming from an alien health care system and written in a form which is difficult to understand. Such theories are dismissed as inapplicable to the British NHS. However even those few theories which do originate in the UK have had limited success. How many people, reading this can identify the compononts of Roper, Logan and Tierney's (1990) work and actually use these, regularly in their practice? The answer, which is easy to predict, is based on a set of assumptions cherished by practitioners. First of all it is assumed that theory is generated by academics; that it is the product of a rarefied world far removed from practice. It therefore follows that practitioners cannot develop theory themselves. This book challenges these assumptions. It highlights the need for practitioners to get involved, to question, to criticize and above all to generate theory from practice, using the language of practice because the 'practice theorist has no illusions about what nursing actually is' (Tolley 1995).

SUMMARY

The aim of this chapter has been to help you explore different meta-paradigms or explanations of the nature of nursing. In doing so the chapter has emphasized the importance of theory in clarifying the role of the profession within the market economy of the health service. If we, as nurses cannot state clearly to purchasers, what nursing can contribute to health care, then they are unlikely to buy our services.

Theory gives a focus to both education and practice development. However this role is undermined by a perceived gap between theory and practice. There is no single or indeed simple explanation for this gap. It is probable that a combination of elements in all three analyses presented here contributes to the problem. Despite this, theory has a central role to play in your practice and this will be explored in the following chapters.

REFERENCES

Carper, B. (1978) Fundamental patterns of knowing in nursing. *Advances in Nursing Science* 1 (1), 13–23.

Chalmers, A. (1982) *What is this thing called science?* 2nd edn, Open University Press, Buckingham.

Chinn, P. and Kramer, M. (1991) *Theory and nursing: a systematic approach*, 3rd edn, Mosby Year Book, St Louis.

Chinn, P. and Kramer, M. (1995) *Theory and nursing: a systematic approach*, 4th edn, Mosby Year Book, St Louis.

Clifford, C. (1993) The clinical role of the nurse teacher in the United Kingdom. *Journal of Advanced Nursing* 18, 281–289.

Cochran, L., Ambutas, S., Buckley, J., D'Arco, S., Donovan, M., Fruth, R., Monico, L. and Scherubel, J. (1989) The Unification model: a collaborative effort. *Nursing Connections* 2 (1), 5–17.

Cook, S. (1991) Mind the theory/practice gap in nursing. *Journal of Advanced Nursing* 16, 1462–1469.

Crotty, M. and Butterworth, T. (1992) The emerging role of the nurse teacher in Project 2000 programmes in England: a literature review. *Journal of Advanced Nursing* 17, 1377–1387.

Dale, A. (1994) The theory–theory gap: the challenge for nurse teachers. *Journal of Advanced Nursing* 20, 521–524.

Dearmun, A. (1993) Reflections of the lecturer practitioner role. *Paediatric Nursing* February, 5 (1), 26–28.

Draper, P. (1990) The development of theory in British Nursing: current position and future prospects. *Journal of Advanced Nursing* 15, 12–15.

Fawcett, J. (1989) *Analysis and evaluation of conceptual models of nursing*, 2nd edn, FA Davis, Philadelphia.

Fawcett, J. (1995) *Analysis and evaluation of conceptual models of nursing*, 3rd edn, FA Davis, Philadelphia.

Fairbrother, P. and Ford, S. (1996) *Mapping the territory: lecturer practitioners in Trent region*. Research Report No 1. Post Graduate Research Centre, University of Sheffield.

Ferguson, K. and Jinks, A. (1994) Integrating what is taught with what is practised in the nursing curriculum: a multi-dimensional model. *Journal of Advanced Nursing* 20, 687–695.

Khadim, N. and Wafer, M. (1993) Bridging the education/practice gap: the Tameside experience. *Journal of Clinical Nursing* 2, 265–267.

Lathlean, J. (1992) The contribution of lecturer-practitioners to theory and practice in nursing. *Journal of Clinical Nursing* 1 (5), 237–242.

Lathlean, J. (1995) *The implementation of lecturer practitioner roles in nursing*. Ashdale Press.

McGee, P. (1993) Developing a model for theatre nursing. *British Journal of Nursing* 2 (5), 262–266.

Menzies, I. (1970) *The use of social systems as a defence against anxiety*. Tavistock Institute for Human Relations, London.

Miller, A. (1985) The relationship between nursing theory and nursing practice. *Journal of Advanced Nursing* 10, 417–424.

Roper, N., Logan, W. and Tierney, A. (1990) *The elements of nursing*, 3rd edn, Churchill Livingstone, Edinburgh.

Royal College of Nursing (1983) *The preparation and education of teachers of nursing*, Royal College of Nursing, London.

Sweeney, N. (1994) A concept analysis of personal knowledge: application to nurse education. *Journal of Advanced Nursing* 20, 917–924.

Tolley, K. (1995) Theory from practice: is this a reality? *Journal of Advanced Nursing* 21, 184–190.

United Kingdom Central Council for Nursing, Midwifery and Health Visiting (1994) *The future of professional practice – the Council's standards for education and practice following registration*, UKCC, London.

White, R. (1985) Political regulators in British nursing. *In:* White, R. (ed.) Political issues in nursing: past present and future, Vol. 1, John Wiley and Sons, Chichester.

Woodrow, P. (1994) Role of the lecturer practitioner 1. *British Journal of Nursing* 3 (11), 571–575.

The person | 4

THE CONCEPT OF THE PERSON

In the previous chapter we examined two explanations of nursing provided by Carper (1978) and Fawcett (1995). The four chapters in this book will explore Fawcett's (1995) ideas in more detail. This particular chapter will look at 'the person' who, according to Fawcett, is the recipient of our nursing care and who may be an individual, a family or a group (Fawcett 1989). The term 'person' is preferred by nurse theorists on the grounds that it is sufficiently broad to embrace all possible recipients. In contrast terms such as 'client' and 'patient' reflect particular groups or classifications of persons.

This chapter will examine the notion of personhood and some the attributes of it, such as individuality and autonomy. The views of several nurse theorists will be put forward in order to help you consider how the recipients of care are regarded in your field of practice and how you see them. The object is to help you question what you do every day and consequently develop your own approach to nursing.

Exercise 4.1 The nature of the person

What concepts and ideas can be included under the heading of 'person?' Spend a few minutes brainstorming this.

Exercises

To begin with we need to consider who or what we think a person is (Fig. 4.1). A person is a human being. Certain attributes, such as personality, ability, intelligence, interests and preferences, demonstrate the uniqueness of that person; that she or he is different from any other. Other attributes show that the person lives in relationships with other people – as a partner, parent, child and has other roles related to work and social activities. Each person is a member of a cultural group which provides an identifiable way of life (Allan 1982). Culture determines how the individual lives; for example, in terms of cooking styles, clothing and types of housing. More importantly it provides the person with values, attitudes and beliefs which influence:

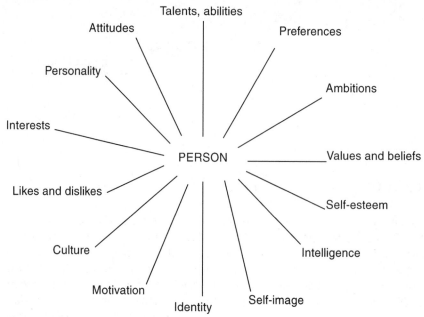

Fig. 4.1 The concept of the person.

- Perceptions of and responses to others.
- A sense of identity and self-concept.
- Daily life, give meaning to it and motivate behaviour.
  (Herberg 1989, Holland 1993).

Culture is learned through socialization (Cooke and Rousseau 1988). An individual's first culture is learned within the family and it becomes an integral part of who that person is. Through school, employment and other settings, the individual is exposed to other cultures, other ways of doing things. Thus the child meets the culture of the school, learns the values and attitudes which the school promotes. In response the child adapts his or her own values and behaviour in order to fit in and contribute to the way of life in the school. Each individual moves through several cultures in the course of a day and is both influenced by and has an influence upon them all.

Culture is therefore a dynamic concept in that the individual is changed by it but also is able to bring about changes within it. Socialization brings about changes in the person as she or he learns a culture but that culture is constantly modified by his or her unique personal characteristics and the setting in which the individual has to function. Cultures have to adapt and change in order to survive (McGee 1992).

THE PERSON AS A RECIPIENT OF NURSING

If all persons are unique in some way, then so is each patient. Nurses constantly emphasize the importance of individualized care, whilst at the same time applying uniform approaches to care delivery right across an

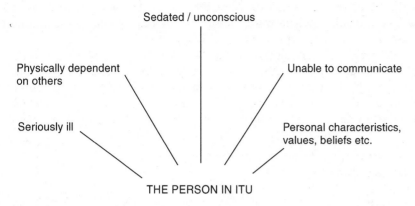

Fig. 4.2 The person in ITU.

organization. This not only suppresses individual care but also ignores the specific needs of patient groups. Figures 4.2 and 4.3 show how persons differ depending on their health/illness status. The person receiving care in ITU (Fig. 4.2) is likely to be completely dependent on nursing and medical staff and be unable to communicate. However this person remains an individual human being irrespective of the level of dependency involved.

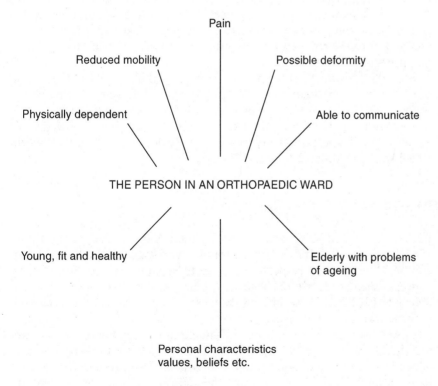

Fig. 4.3 The person in an orthopaedic ward.

Staff therefore have to ensure that they act in the best interests of this person and take into account factors such as age, gender, religion and personal preferences which may all influence care.

The person in an orthopaedic ward (Fig. 4.3) may be seen quite differently. A young person with a sports injury for example, may be regarded as physically dependent but otherwise fit and healthy, well able to communicate and thus easily frustrated by having to stay in bed. Alternatively, an older adult may have both physical and intellectual/sensory impairments which affect communication and decision making.

Discussion

Discussion Topic 4.1

Are there different patient groups within your practice area? For example, in an ENT ward you might have dental patients, oncology patients and emergency admissions. How would you describe the people in each of these groups? What are their characteristics?

If we are to truly acknowledge the individuality of patients we should start by emphasizing the ways in which patient groups differ and make those differences explicit. To impose a single model of care across all the working environments within an organization creates a situation in which nurses are forced to squeeze their patients into a framework in which they do not fit. Clear indicators of the differences between client groups should be helpful in enabling nursing teams to determine the best approach to care and justify to their managers why a blanket application of any model is inappropriate.

Secondly, it is worthwhile spending some time thinking about the nature of our particular patient/client groups to ensure that we see them appropriately. Do we see them as people like ourselves and thus worthy of the respect and dignity we would like extended to us? If so, how do we demonstrate this respect; what are we actually doing in our place of work which shows respect for patients/clients?

RESPECT FOR PERSONS

Respect is a moral obligation to benefit others and a human right (Gillon 1985, Browne 1993). It therefore does not have to be earned and we cannot choose those we will respect. We have to separate respect from other concepts such as regard for those in authority or those who have achieved (McGee 1994). This is difficult because some ideas are very closely entwined with those of respect.

Low self-esteem or a negative self-image can affect whether or not an individual can give respect to others. Thus the ability to respect others depends to some extent on respect for the self. A lack of respect for the self, invites a similar lack of respect from others. Respect also has an association with reciprocity in that individuals who feel respected by others also feel able to give respect in return (Sugitherajah 1994).

In nursing, respect permeates everything we do. If we do not respect those we nurse 'there is little point in what we do. Nursing without respect dehumanizes patients' (McGee 1994). Respect is demonstrated by approaching others as equals in the nurse–patient relationship. Browne (1993) suggests three ways in which nurses can show respect:

1. Non-verbal signals such as facial expression.
2. General courtesy and the active use of a communication style which seeks to avoid offence.
3. Acting in a way which recognizes the patient's/client's rights to be informed and make decisions. This must be afforded even though the nurse may disagree with the patient/client and even when the nurse has to point out to the patient/client the potentially harmful consequences arising from a particular decision.

Respect then is about how we treat the recipients of our nursing on a day to day basis; about placing ourselves on the same level as those we care for. Numerous reports and enquiries would suggest that this does not always happen; that the recipients of care are frequently treated as less than human. Everyone is appalled when the dramatic stories hit the headlines and says 'It couldn't happen where I work because . . .' but consider this. In the days before Project 2000, student nurses were required to take an examination in which they provided care for a patient for a span of duty during which they were observed by an assessor. I assessed students on many occasions. Among those I failed were a student who placed a patient on the commode in the middle of the ward without drawing the screens. Another student wiped a wet chair with the patient's pyjama jacket and then dressed him in the same jacket. A third student looked aghast when instructed to ask a patient what he wanted to do that morning. None of these students thought that what they had done mattered a jot. Their actions were not important in the real work of nursing. I would argue that if these things can happen when nurses are trying to do things correctly, because they are being observed, what they get up to the rest of the time must be a matter of grave concern.

It also suggests that some nurses do not see the recipients of their care as people like themselves but as people less than themselves, for whom much lower standards apply. Such nurses would not use a commode without the screen being drawn but think it is alright for the patients to do so. The students I assessed were not aware of the implications of what they were doing and did not intend any harm. They would probably be horrified if anyone accused them of abusing patients, so where did they learn to behave like this? There is no easy answer to this question but maybe some of them learned, not from us, because we set out to give the best care we can, but because of us or more correctly, because of our professional values.

Discussion

Discussion Topic 4.2

What values can you identify in your practice? What, for example, is considered important? Is there rivalry between staff groups?

As a profession nurses tend to value getting the work done, preferably as quickly as possible. The night staff, for example, do more and more to show the day staff how efficient they are. Any ward nurse who has not finished washing patients by coffee time is termed 'slow'. It is hardly surprising that, in order to meet the impossible deadlines we set, some nurses cut corners. More seriously, we have allowed ourselves to be convinced by the argument that the delivery of direct care by a qualified nurse is an expensive waste of resources. As a result we have allowed less qualified and maybe sometimes less able staff to go their own way. The result is that some have gradually slid downwards.

It is therefore not enough to say that I, as a practitioner, see my patients/clients in a particular way. We need to identify how our colleagues see them. There must be agreement among the various nursing team members so that all work together. In addition we should ask whether the nurses' views of the recipients of their care matches the views of the recipients themselves. The demonstration of respect is a two-way process. Patients have a right to respect as human beings but nurses are human beings too and entitled to receive respect in return. Moreover both parties need to feel respected by the other and a growing number of reports suggest that the reciprocal element of respect between nurses and patients is breaking down. Nurses in some settings report routinely experiencing violence and aggression (Knight 1997) which suggests that either patients no longer respect them or that professional- and self-esteem is so low that nurses no longer feel respected.

NURSE THEORISTS' VIEWS OF THE PERSON

It is helpful at this point to look at what has been published by other theorists regarding the nature of the person. These views of the person are all quite general and do not relate to any specific care setting, but they offer ideas which you may find helpful in developing your own opinions.

In examining these views we can establish a number of commonalities between theorists, as well as differences of opinion. The person is seen as an individual who is separate from, but who interacts with others and the environment. Peplau and Roper stress the uniqueness of each individual which is apparent in his/her behaviour. King and Roy see the individual as being composed of systems but their opinions vary on the nature of those systems. In particular they emphasize the importance of systems in helping the individual adapt and cope with external stimuli. In contrast, Roper sees the individual as a whole and pursuing a set of

Exercise 4.2

Compare and contrast the differing views of the person provided by the following nurse theorists.

Peplau
The person is an organism with physical, social and particularly psychological needs. Needs create tension and the person always strives to reduce this by engaging in specific behaviours which will meet specific needs (Simpson 1991). Each person is unique and will not react in the same way as any other. Each is also capable of growing and changing (Carey *et al.* 1989).

Nightingale
The person/patient is the recipient of the nurse's care and as such is passive. However, given the appropriate environment, the patient has the power to deal with disease (Nightingale 1860/1969).

Roper
The person is an individual who pursues the complex process of living in a unique manner through a number of activities. These activities are influenced by the person's place on the lifespan continuum, physical, psychological, sociocultural, environmental and politico-economic factors and the degree of independence/dependence which the individual has (Roper *et al.* 1990).

King
The person is a set of systems which are:

- personal including perception (how we experience the world around us), sense of self, growth and development, body image, personal space, and time;
- interpersonal including how we interact with others and social roles. Interactions can produce stress;
- social which are structured to achieve goals. Social systems are based around people e.g. family, values and needs, technology.

The person has three fundamental health care needs; information, prevention of illness and care when unable to help himself (King 1981).

Roy
The person is a complex, adaptive system made up of bio-psycho-social subsystems in constant interaction with the changing environment. The environment bombards the individual with three types of stimuli:

- focal – stimuli which the individual immediately confronts;
- contextual – which occur alongside focal stimuli;
- residual – other factors such as past experience.

The individual reacts to these stimuli through adaptation in one or more of the four modes which are:

- physiological;
- role performance, i.e. social role change;
- self-concept;
- interdependence, i.e. changes in relationships with others.

Each subsystem tries to maintain harmony in the body and with the outside environment (Roy 1984).

activities whilst being influenced by a number of external factors. Thus the majority of these theorists portray the individual as actively involved with people and the environment in order to maintain internal harmony. The exception is Nightingale who is the only theorist here to use the term 'patient' and who sees that person in a rather more passive role. However even she acknowledges that the patient has some innate power to cope with illness.

The different views of Nightingale can be linked to the society and period in which she wrote. In particular we have to be aware of different notions about the nature of the individual. In tracing the history of this concept the best summary is be found in Williams (1961) who argues that in mediaeval thought this word meant 'indivisible' and was used in Christian theology to explain the Holy Trinity. Gradually its use was extended to describe membership of a secular group. An individual was defined by membership of a particular social group; peasants, craftsmen, knights. Our modern concept of the individual began to emerge around the early seventeenth century, under the influence of philosophers such as Descartes, with 'the abstraction of the individual from the complex of relationships by which he had hitherto normally been defined' (Williams 1961). From then on, the concept of the individual continued to evolve. With the development of industrialization came new debates about the nature of the person, particularly that of whether humans were a type of machine. Added to this was the concept of 'class', that 'the individual relates to his society through his class' (Williams 1961) which will cause the individual to think and act in particular ways. Thus Nightingale may be said to be a product of her class, regarding the sick, and indeed nurses, in particular ways. In summary, her thinking pre-dates many of the influences, especially Freud, which we have incorporated into our view of the individual and the person.

INDIVIDUALITY

Most of the theorists we have examined in this chapter clearly value the modern concept of the individual and in following their ideas we are asked to recognize that no two people will react to illness or changes to their health in the same way. Consequently we have to take these individual differences into account when we plan nursing care. However, we have also to consider the extent to which we can realistically do so. How many ward/unit philosophies state that nursing teams provide individualized, holistic care, when in fact they cannot do so? Yet in stating such an aim they raise expectations which cannot be met and then feel threatened when patients complain.

Valuing the concept of the individual reflects the norms of western society in which the individual is expected to exercise autonomy which involves taking charge of one's own life. This view of the individual was certainly not present in Nightingale's era and it is important to recognize that, even today, other societies may have different ideas. For example

Margolis (1993) describes the socialization experienced by former East Germans who stated that

> we were brought up in a collective. The aim was not to be an individual and catch the attention of others. There was a saying in the GDR 'From the me to the we'. There was never an I, just the we.

Margolis offers us an extreme example but even in our own society it can be difficult for people to function as separate individuals. The

> . . . dominant quest in our culture for extreme individualism, the quest to be in charge of one's own life and control all the options, including feelings and responses to events. (Benner and Wrubel 1989)

runs counter to the realities of life for many people. This is particularly so for those who are dependent on others because 'from a place of care, the person can neither claim complete autonomy nor be the absolute source of all meaning' (Benner and Wrubel 1989). Being with people, participating in relationships, caring for others all interfere with the pursuit of extreme individuality. Even if it were possible to relinquish all ties and become completely independent of everyone, the result would be 'negative freedom' which deprives the person of the positive freedom to choose and act (Benner and Wrubel 1989).

Discussion Topic 4.3

What, in your opinion, do nurses mean when they talk about individualized care? Is individualized care possible in your practice area? What factors affect the provision and delivery of individualized care in your practice area?

Discussion

The concept of the individual is linked therefore with that of autonomy which is a central issue in health care. Individuals are regarded as self-governing in other aspects of their lives; able to deal with problems and make decisions. Health problems are no different to any other in terms of the difficulties they create. It is illogical to say that an individual who can deal with other problems cannot deal with health problems. Consequently individuals are deemed capable of making decisions about health in the same way as they would decide which car to buy or which film to see. This is an important and valuable aspect of our health care system. Upholding the rights of individuals to make decisions about their lives is a central element in demonstrating respect for them and in accepting both individual and cultural differences.

AUTONOMY

Autonomy is not a single entity. Personal autonomy is that exercised by the individual who is able to take charge of his or her own life (Seedhouse

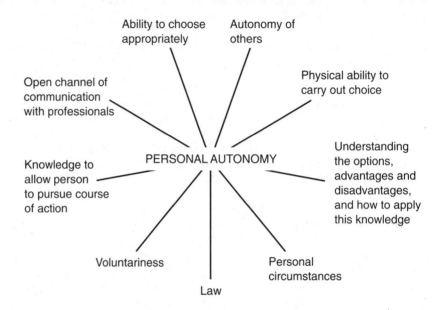

Fig. 4.4 Influences on personal autonomy (based on Seedhouse 1988, Bandman and Bandman 1990, Jensen and Mooney 1990).

1988). In this context autonomy is seen as a basic right and responsibility for decisions is placed solely on the individual. In reality this form of autonomy is constantly modified by a number of factors (Fig. 4.4) which in the health care setting are first and foremost likely to be affected by the patient's illness (Seedhouse 1988, Bandman and Bandman 1990, Jensen and Mooney 1990).

For example, Mrs Green is involved in a car accident. She sustains a fractured femur and some other injuries. After the accident it is likely that others will take charge of her and take her to hospital thus compromising the principle of voluntariness (that she has gone there of her own free will). Her ability to make decisions is further modified (Fig. 4.4) by:

- Pain.
- The degree of openness in communication shown by professionals who may be overworked and stressed.
- Personal circumstances, for example whether there is anyone at home who might be willing to provide care, plus their views about what should happen.
- The amount of knowledge she has about her injuries, her condition and the possible treatments. This includes knowledge of bone structure and healing as well as respiratory function and the techniques which might be used to repair the injuries.
- Her understanding of the options available, the pros and cons of these, and which would be the most appropriate in the circumstances.

- Her ability to choose appropriately.
- Her ability to carry out her choice especially if it does not conform to what the professionals wish to provide.
- The law, for example, if she was found to have a raised level of blood alcohol whilst driving the car.

Thus decision making by the individual becomes a complex process involving interaction with others who are also exercising their autonomy. If all these individuals make the same decision there will be no conflict. However if Mrs Green makes a decision which the professionals think is incorrect then conflict is inevitable, especially as she is not able to get up and leave.

It can be argued that this form of autonomy facilitates the development of the market economy in that

> . . . the prime strategy for rationing health care that emerges from this principle of autonomy is that of the private market. The informed rational consumer chooses on the demand side of the market and independently on the supply side, the producers respond. (Jensen and Mooney 1990)

To illustrate this, in everyday life, if an individual wants to buy a washing machine s/he might obtain a copy of the *Which?* report, consult with friends, phone a number of companies to compare prices and so on. In the end the individual would make a decision based on what could be afforded and the most suitable machine. If this process is applied to health care, services are developed to increase the range of consumer choice and the individual 'shops around' for the best deal. This in turn allows for services to be rationed to those who can afford them. The problem is that, as we have seen, in an emergency situation, such shopping around is not possible.

Discussion

Discussion Topic 4.4

Choose two patients from your practice area and critically examine the factors which may affect their personal autonomy.

Moreover if Mrs Green chooses to reject the professionals' opinions on what should be done to help her; and if professionals give her only what she wants, as opposed to what she really needs, then their integrity is compromised (May 1995). Individual autonomy, whilst desirable, must be balanced by respect for the autonomy of others and serve needs before wants (Seedhouse 1988). This *relativistic autonomy* recognizes that there are no absolute rights or standards. Thus individual circumstances can be taken into account when making decisions. Individuals are still free to make choices but professionals are also free to contribute their perspectives so that decision making is informed by dialogue and negotiation (Jenson and Mooney 1990).

In nursing practice this is probably the form of autonomy most often used. For example, after surgery a patient may have a painful wound and so does not wish to get out of bed. The nurse recognizes that by allowing the patient to exercise personal autonomy, a thrombosis or a chest infection may occur. Through the exercise of relativistic autonomy the nurse is able to explain why getting up is so important and to negotiate with the patient about how this might be achieved.

Relativistic autonomy allows the individual and the nurse equal power but it also allows the nurse to influence the amount of autonomy the individual has (Seedhouse 1988). Thus autonomy can be created, for example, by ensuring that the individual is pain free, respecting Mrs Green's point of view and facilitating an open channel of communication between her and the nurse. Autonomy can be increased by, for example, the nurse providing information for the patient and making an effort to negotiate a settlement which is mutually satisfactory. Autonomy can thus be enhanced through mutual trust and respect between the nurse and the individual or diminished by the use of dogmatic, authoritarian attitudes.

The difficulty with this type of autonomy is that nurses and other health professionals can end up acting as the gatekeepers of the knowledge which the patient needs to participate in dialogue and negotiation. In such circumstances communication becomes one way and the patient is not informed of the options or given any room for manoeuvre. Passivity is encouraged and the professionals do what they think is best (Jensen and Mooney 1990).

POWER

Autonomy therefore has a strong relationship with power. In recent literature, professional power seems to be regarded as a bad thing. Illych (1978) compares professionals to gangsters running a protection racket by convincing people that they had needs which only the professionals could supply. Sines (1994) argues that

> ... in keeping with the total institutional model, some of our present hospitals continue to appear to be characterized by a world divided in two, where managers dominate the front line workers and where staff dominate their clients in turn. (Sines 1994)

The recent health service reforms have also contributed to challenging the wisdom that professionals always know best.

Gilbert (1995) proposes that some forms of power are dependent on conflict. The one who wins the battles gains power. Other forms of power serve to prevent conflict by 'operating to produce and shape the perceptions, cognitions and preferences of people in such a way that they accept social practices, and their role, as the natural way' (Gilbert 1995). Consequently people do not, or are not encouraged to, consider alternatives. However, power can also be defined positively, for example in personal terms. Personal growth leads to personal power and subsequent freedom from oppression. Personal power can be collectivized so that if a group or community work together they will have greater power (Gilbert 1995).

The problem with all these explanations is that none captures the multifaceted nature of power or the complexity of human interaction. They do however raise questions about the nature and exercise of power in nursing. In this analysis there are many variations. For example, Keen and Malby (1992) argue that, in managerial terms nurses have missed the power boat because they do not have 'a clear sense of what they have to offer' (Keen and Malby 1992). Harrison and Pollitt (1994) appear to disagree stating that while the introduction of general management took away the right of nurses to be managed by a member of the same profession, nurses were 'quick to capitalise upon Griffith's emphasis on the impact of health care upon the patient' (Harrison and Pollitt 1994) and consequently the careers of nurse managers 'overall career opportunities will be no worse than before Griffiths' (Harrison and Pollitt 1994). Thus nursing can accrue power through becoming managerialized.

In the arena of patient care, Hewison (1995a) showed how nurses use language to exert power over patients; to give instructions, persuade or control patient activity. He also identified a category of interaction which he called 'terms of endearment' in which nurses exerted power through caring terms such as 'good girl', 'pet' or 'sweetie'. It comes as something of a surprise to find that patients engaged in exactly the same behaviour even though this is 'only to a degree, the control they (patients) exert is still related to the tasks of the nurses' (Hewison, personal correspondence). Clearly power in the nurse–patient relationship is not entirely one-sided.

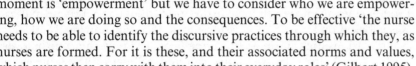

Reading Suggestion 4.1

Read Hewison, A. (1995) Nurses' power in interaction with patients. *Journal of Advanced Nursing* 21, 75–82.
    Listen to conversations between nurses and patients. Identify examples of the use of language to exert power and control over others.
    Which examples enhance patient care and why?

Reading

In considering power in our nursing practice we therefore have to consider what types of power we have and how we exercise it. The buzz word at the moment is 'empowerment' but we have to consider who we are empowering, how we are doing so and the consequences. To be effective 'the nurse needs to be able to identify the discursive practices through which they, as nurses are formed. For it is these, and their associated norms and values, which nurses then carry with them into their everyday roles' (Gilbert 1995).

WHO IS A PERSON?

Having considered some of the conceptual elements of the person as defined by nurse theorists, we should also examine 'person' as a term. There are several opposing views of the person which are briefly outlined here:

The mechanistic/reductionist view

The person is passive, an object, subject to and responsive to stimuli. The person functions in the same way as a machine and can therefore be subdivided into elementary component parts in order to explain how the machine works. Thus the mind is separated from the body which is further divided into systems. This view of the person is used in certain care settings. For example intensive care where the emphasis is on bringing stability to certain body systems and day surgery units with a very fast turnover in which there is little opportunity to focus on individuals in detail. However, in concentrating on particular body systems or operations it is possible to lose sight of the individual and treat the condition rather than the person.

The phenomenological view

The person is not an object; is active rather than passive; has an internal locus of control. Moreover the person exists within a social context and cannot be separated from it. Rather than dividing the person, the phenomenologist view focuses on holism, that the whole is greater that the sum of the parts (Chinn and Kramer 1995).

The person is regarded as an intelligent being who can reason and reflect. The person is self-conscious and self-aware not only in the present but over time; 'a thinking intelligent being, that has reason and reflection, and considers itself, the same thinking thing, in different times and places; which it does only by that consciousness which is inseparable from thinking and seems to be essential to it; it being impossible for anyone to perceive without perceiving that he does perceive' (Locke 1976).

This view of the person pervades much of nursing theory and reflects what most nurses will say they strive to achieve in their care. Holism seeks to provide better quality health care in a more humane manner. It is also in tune with societal changes which have undermined the passivity of patients and encouraged them to question professionals. However, given the realities of nursing practice, one has to ask whether holistic approaches to care are simply superficial gloss spread over more traditional systems of delivering services. Nurses are encouraged to get to know their patients through assessments which include questions about very private matters. This is based on a number of assumptions: that the individual welcomes such intrusions; that it is possible to really get to know someone in a very short space of time; that the nurse can and will act on the information received (May 1995).

Discussion

Discussion Topic 4.5

Which view of the person is most used in your practice area and why?

The human being view

All persons are essentially human beings. To distinguish between the two is to suggest that there are human beings who are persons because they are self-aware and intelligent (Locke 1976) and human beings who are non-persons because they cannot meet certain specified criteria (Allmark 1994). As nurses we have to acknowledge that a good many of our patients, either permanently or at some time, will fail to meet these criteria. If nursing concerns itself only with persons as defined by Locke then it is available only to a specific sector of society. We are then faced with the question of what happens to the non-persons in terms of nursing and health care. In the context of the rationing of resources, the distinctions between persons and humans facilitates decisions about who should receive care: 'who should have priority for being helped to live and those who are valued as less important' (Bandman and Bandman 1990).

It is evident that none of these views gives us a comprehensive definition of what a person is, nor do they consistently help us as nurses. We therefore need to develop definitions of the person which are sufficiently broad to enable us to met the needs of many different subgroups of persons and provide nursing care in a morally acceptable way. These definitions must help us not only in dealing with current situations but also in considering the future of individual persons. In doing so we must examine the potential of individual persons and ensure that 'the achievement of a desired potential in an individual should not decrease the amount of future potentials open to that individual that might enhance her existence' (Seedhouse 1988). Moreover these potentials should not be achieved at the expense of 'avoidable dwarfing in other people' (Seedhouse 1988).

SUMMARY

Fawcett's (1995) explanation of nursing states that one of the important elements of professional concern, is the person. This chapter has examined some of the issues surrounding the concept of the person who is both a unique individual, a social and cultural being. The person is essentially a human being because all other definitions potentially exclude certain groups of people. The views of a number of nurse theorists have been considered in relation to what they have to say about the nature of the recipient of nursing activities.

Most modern theorists tend to see the person in holistic terms as someone able to interact with others and the environment. In this context all persons are entitled to unconditional respect as a basic human right. Respect must permeate nursing activities at all levels because without it, patients are dehumanized and abused. Nurses also deserve respect from patients in that they are also human beings, and should not have to tolerate violence and abuse.

A part of demonstrating respect lies in exercising autonomy in a manner which enables others to remain in charge of their lives even when they are very dependent. Nurses have a role to play in increasing the autonomy of patients. However, it would seem that the current vogue for patient autonomy may actually have hidden agendas with regard to the development of a purchaser–provider economy and the rationing of health care services.

Whilst the holistic view of the person is both practical and desirable, the extent to which it can be implemented can vary. We have to look more honestly at the realities of what is happening in practice. In acute care settings, much of what nurses do is still based on the mechanistic view of the person because that person is either unconscious or is in and out of the health care setting so rapidly that the opportunity for any kind of meaningful interpersonal and therapeutic relationship is severely limited. In some instances the nature of the client may make holistic care impossible. In others the mechanistic view may be used initially to deal with an emergency situation and a more holistic view applied as the person's condition improves.

Reading

Reading Suggestion 4.2

Henry, C. and Tuxill, A. (1987) Concept of the person: introduction to the health professionals' curriculum. *Journal of Advanced Nursing* 12, 245–249.

Johns, C. (1990) Autonomy of primary nurses: the need to both facilitate and limit autonomy. *Journal of Advanced Nursing* 15, 886–894.

Philpot, T. (1994) The ethics of smoke free zones: an exploration of the implications and effectiveness of a non-smoking policy as a health promotion strategy in the context of an orthopaedic trauma ward. *Journal of Clinical Nursing* 3, 307–311.

Exercises

Exercise 4.3 Developing your own approach to care: the person

Either by yourself or with a small group, discuss the following questions and record your answers on flip charts.

1. How do you see the persons who receive care from you?
2. How do your colleagues see these persons?
3. What factors influence how you see these people?

REFERENCES

Allan, S. (1982) Perhaps a seventh person. *In:* Husband, C. (ed.) *Race in Britain*, Hutchinson University Library, London.

Allmark, P. (1994) An argument against the use of the concept of 'persons' in health care ethics. *Journal of Advanced Nursing* 19, 29–35.

Bandman, E. and Bandman, B. (1990) *Nursing ethics through the lifespan*, 2nd edn, Prentice Hall, London.

Benner, P. and Wrubel, J. (1989) *The primacy of caring: stress and coping in health and illness*, Addison Wesley, Menlo Park Calif.

Browne, A. (1993) A conceptual clarification of respect. *Journal of Advanced Nursing* 18, 211–217.

Carper, B. (1978) Fundamental patterns of knowing in nursing. *Advances in Nursing Science* 1 (1), 13–23.

Carey, E., Noll, J., Rasmussen, L., Searcy, B. and Stark, N. (1989) Hildegard E. Peplau. *In:* Marriner-Twomey, A. (ed.) *Nursing theorists and their work*, 2nd edn, CV Mosby, St Louis.

Chinn, P and Kramer, M. (1995) *Theory and Nursing*, 4th edn, Mosby Year Book, St Louis.

Cooke, R. and Rousseau, D. (1988) Behavioural norms and expectations. A quantitative approach to the assessment of organizational culture. *Group and Organizational Studies* September 13 (3), 245–273.

Fawcett, J. (1989) *Analysis and evaluation of conceptual models of nursing*, 2nd edn, FA Davis, Philadelphia.

Fawcett, J. (1995) *Analysis and evaluation of conceptual models of nursing*, 3rd edn, FA Davis, Philadelphia.

Gilbert, T. (1995) Nursing: empowerment and the problem of power. *Journal of Advanced Nursing* 21, 865–871.

Gillon, R (1985) *Philosophical medical ethics*. John Wiley and Sons, Chichester.

Harrison, S. and Pollitt, C. (1994) *Controlling health professionals. The future of work and organization in the NHS*. Open University Press, Buckingham.

Herberg, P. (1989) Theoretical foundations of transcultural nursing. *In:* Boyle, J. and Andrews, M. (eds) *Transcultural concepts in nursing care*, Scott, Foresman/ Little Brown College Division, Glenview, Illinois.

Hewison, A. (1995) Nurses' power in interaction with patients. *Journal of Advanced Nursing*. 21, 75–82.

Holland, C. (1993) An ethnographic study of nursing culture as an exploration for determining the existence of a system of ritual. *Journal of Advanced Nursing* 18, 1461–1470.

Illych, I. (1978) *Disabling professions*, Marion Boyars, London.

Jensen, U. and Mooney, G. (1990) Changing values: autonomy and paternalism and health care. *In*: Jensen, U. and Mooney, G. (eds) *Changing values in medical and health care decision making*, John Wiley and Sons, Chichester.

Keen, J. and Malby, R. (1992) Nursing power and practice in United Kingdom National Health Service. *Journal of Advanced Nursing* 17, 863–870.

King, I. (1981) *A theory for nursing: systems, concepts process*, John Wiley and Sons, New York.

Knight, K. (1997) Fear and violence: my typical night in casualty. *The Times*, 23 May 1997, p. 8.

Locke, J. (1976) *An essay concerning human understanding*, Oxford University Press, Oxford.

McGee, P. (1992) *Teaching transcultural care: a guide for teachers of nursing and health professions*, Chapman and Hall, London.

McGee, P. (1994) The concept of respect in nursing. *British Journal of Nursing* 3 (13), 681,683–684.

Margolis, J. (1993) The post-Marxist makeover. *The Sunday Times* 17 October, Style and Travel, p. 11.

May, C. (1995) Patient autonomy and the politics of professional relationships. *Journal of Advanced Nursing* 21, 83–87.

Nightingale, F. (1860/1969) *Notes on nursing: what it is and what it is not.* Dover Publications Inc, New York, First published 1860.

Roy, C. (1984) *Introduction to nursing: an adaptation model*, 2nd edn, Prentice Hall, Englewood Cliffs, New Jersey.

Roper, N., Logan, W. and Tierney, A. (1990) *The elements of nursing*, 3rd edn, Churchill Livingstone, Edinburgh.

Seedhouse, D. (1988) *Ethics: the heart of health care*, John Wiley and Sons, Chichester.

Seedhouse, D. (1991) *Liberating medicine*, John Wiley and Sons, Chichester.

Simpson, H. (1991) *Peplau's model in action*, Macmillan, Houndmills.

Sines, D. (1994) The arrogance of power: a reflection on contemporary mental health nursing practice. *Journal of Advanced Nursing* 20, 894–903.

Sugitherajah, S. (1994) The concept of respect in Asian tradition. *British Journal of Nursing* 3 (14), 739–741.

Williams, R. (1961) *The long revolution*, Penguin Books in association with Chatto and Windus, Harmondsworth.

Health 5

NURSE THEORISTS' VIEWS OF HEALTH

Fawcett (1995) defines health as 'the person's state of well being, which can range from high level wellness to terminal illness' (Fawcett 1995). Within this broad definition, health can be seen by some theorists, such as Newman, as a state of being which incorporates illness (Chinn and Kramer 1991) or as a continuum as described by Roper *et al.* (1990). Figure 5.1 gives an overview of the position of other nurse theorists on health.

Discussion Topic 5.1

Compare and contrast the definitions of health in Figure 5.1.

Which do you agree/disagree with and why?

Discussion

From these definitions it is evident that there is no single definition of health and that, with the exception of Nightingale, health is more than the absence of disease. As with the examination of the nature of the person, Nightingale's ideas must be seen within the context of her time, when many life-threatening illnesses such as cholera were caused by factors in the environment. Attitudes to illness were very different and Nightingale castigates some of these in her writings. For example, people particularly feared the night air as a source of illness but 'what air can we breathe at night but night air? The choice is between pure night air from without and foul night air from within' (Nightingale 1860/1969).

Modern views of health are much broader. Health is not static. It is dynamic, requiring, on the part of the person, some activity such as adaptation (Roy and King) or personal development (Peplau). In this context health is an elusive concept without the certainty of Nightingale's day. In addition we have to consider that these nursing views of health compete with others both interprofessionally and in the political arena. This chapter will examine some of the current models of health, in terms of their usefulness to nursing, with the aim of developing a positive approach to health in your practice.

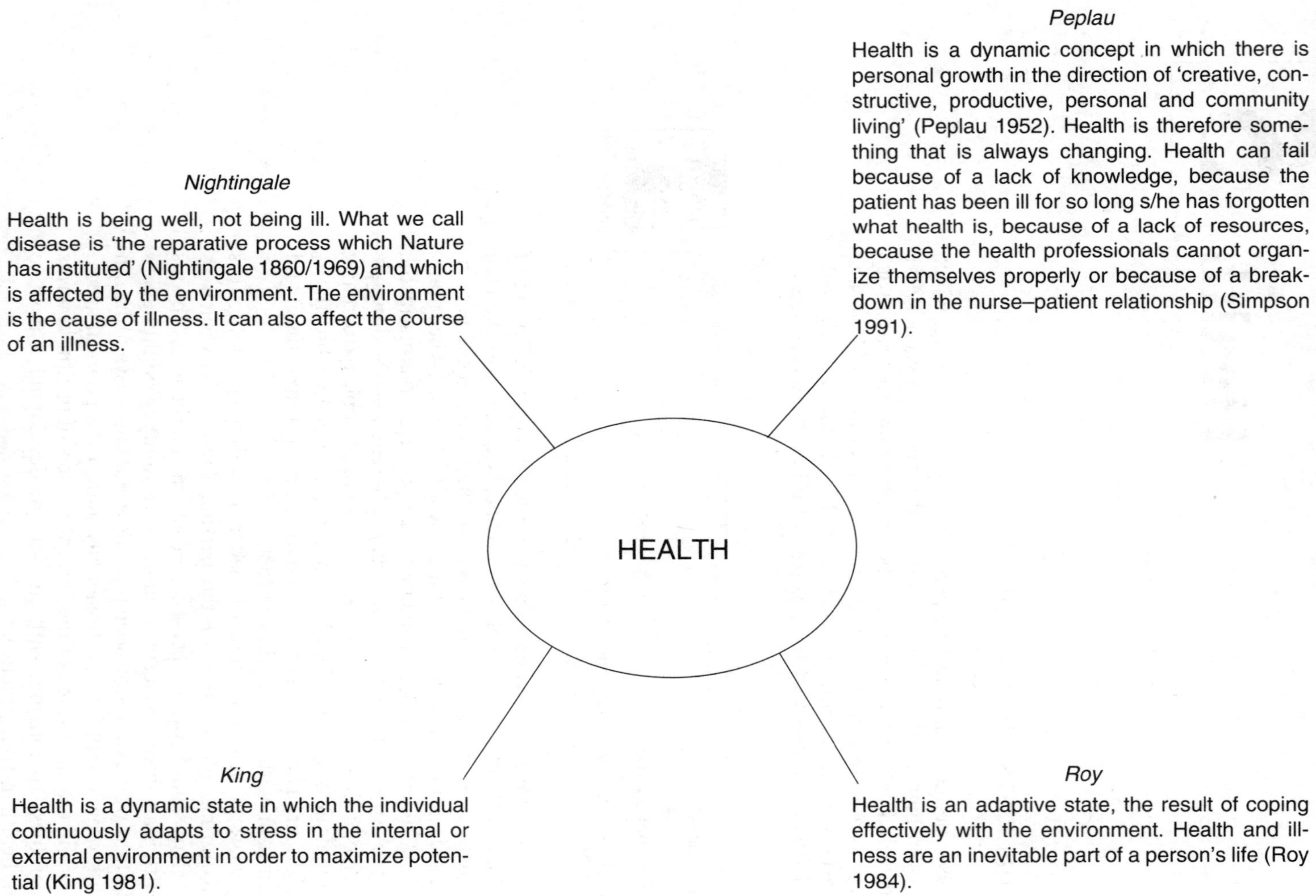

Peplau

Health is a dynamic concept in which there is personal growth in the direction of 'creative, constructive, productive, personal and community living' (Peplau 1952). Health is therefore something that is always changing. Health can fail because of a lack of knowledge, because the patient has been ill for so long s/he has forgotten what health is, because of a lack of resources, because the health professionals cannot organize themselves properly or because of a breakdown in the nurse–patient relationship (Simpson 1991).

Roy

Health is an adaptive state, the result of coping effectively with the environment. Health and illness are an inevitable part of a person's life (Roy 1984).

Nightingale

Health is being well, not being ill. What we call disease is 'the reparative process which Nature has instituted' (Nightingale 1860/1969) and which is affected by the environment. The environment is the cause of illness. It can also affect the course of an illness.

King

Health is a dynamic state in which the individual continuously adapts to stress in the internal or external environment in order to maximize potential (King 1981).

HEALTH

Fig. 5.1 An overview of nursing theorists' views on health.

THE BIOTECHNOLOGICAL MODEL OF HEALTH

This is based on western medicine and the classification of illnesses which it provides. The body is explained in mechanistic terms and there is emphasis on body systems rather than the whole person. Like any other machine the body can develop mechanical faults which can be rectified through the application of biomedical sciences and technology (Beattie 1995, Doyal 1995). Similarly potential faults can be minimized through certain courses of action, in much the same way as you might 'turn over' the engine of a car, if it is left standing for a long period of time, in order to ensure that it will start when needed.

Usefulness to nursing

This model has been extremely successful, for example in dealing with infectious diseases and certain physical abnormalities. Patients undergoing surgery for hip replacement can be seen to have developed a mechanical fault and may arrive in hospital barely able to walk. Surgery, in theory, should correct the fault and enable them to regain mobility. Part of the job satisfaction for nurses in orthopaedic wards lies in facilitating this kind of improvement and much of their knowledge base must centre around helping the patient to gain confidence and become more mobile, whilst at the same time preventing complications. Patients may therefore be said to have attained health when they can walk around the ward unaided, sit down and get up from a chair, get in and out of bed and the bath, and climb the stairs.

However, the idea of mechanical failure does not explain all aspects of health and illness. It does not help us to understand why some bodies are more likely to develop certain faults whilst others do not. Nor does it explain why illness may occur in the mind which cannot be equated to a machine.

We also have to consider the basis of the concept of mechanical fault. Is there an ideal body machine and what is it like? Doyal (1995) argues that the reductionism of this model and the male domination of the medical profession has 'limited its potential either to understand or to ameliorate the ills of both sexes'. Women have suffered from a male-dominated paradigm in which their bodies are compared to those of men. There has been little effort to examine health issues which affect only women. There is little research on how problems which affect both men and women, such as coronary heart disease, might show differences in symptoms and require different treatment strategies (Doyal 1995).

Current health knowledge is therefore homocentric and eurocentric. As such it is potentially, if not actually oppressive (Airhihenbuwa 1995). There has been less attention paid to health problems which have affected pre-dominantly non-white populations such as the haemoglobinopathies. In addition it is recognized that the incidence of conditions such as diabetes is considerably higher among ethnic minority people living in developed countries but the reasons remain largely unexplored (Raymond and

D'Eramo-Melkus 1993). The biotechnological model does not allow for variations which may cross gender or racial boundaries nor does it encourage the nurse to adapt or develop skills to meet the needs of patients in these groups.

Finally this model focuses on the individual to the possible exclusion of others. The emphasis is on either correcting or minimizing the mechanical fault. In the correction mode, the individual's wishes and circumstances are of secondary importance and may be considered only in relation to achieving a successful correction. Their social and cultural contexts are not considered. In the minimizing mode the individual is instructed in a course of action and is expected to follow it. Thus s/he is informed that coronary artery disease can be minimized through specified activities such as a change of diet, exercise and giving up smoking. Having been given this information the individual is expected to assume responsibility for minimizing coronary heart disease in his/her own body machine by following the instructions. Subsequent coronary heart disease can then be said to be the individual's own fault, conveniently ignoring the fact that other factors may be involved (Naidoo 1986) which are outside that person's control.

The biotechnological model is therefore applicable in certain fields of nursing but it is not comprehensive. It offers only a limited explanation of events in terms of health problems and gender divisions. It also ignores the individual as a holistic being who may have particular wishes or needs. Factors which affect an individual's health are not always within his or her control.

THE HEALTH AS A COMMODITY MODEL

This has much in common with the biotechnological model. If the body functions like a machine, and can be looked after in much the same way as a car or tumble dryer, then it is possible to buy in maintenance services. A health mechanic becomes as feasible as a car mechanic. Health is a commodity which can be bought and sold (Benner and Wrubel 1989).

Usefulness to nursing

The strengths and limitations of the biotechnological model apply here but there are additional issues for consideration. First of all health is placed as something outside the self. The individual does not automatically possess it, which could imply that we are all unhealthy unless we spend money on purchasing health. The amount of health we have therefore depends on how much we can afford. If we are purchasing it directly, we expect value for our money, 'instant cures without person effort' (Benner and Wrubel 1989); to be able to complain if the service does not match our expectations, just as we would to any other service contractor and finally to have the sanction of being able to take our custom elsewhere. This may just work in relation to planned surgery. It is possible to envisage shopping around for the best deal on hip replacement. It could also be possible to do the same to obtain care in chronic illness. Emergencies present a different picture challenging the idea that patients can exercise personal autonomy in this way. It is difficult to imagine someone surfing the net for the best coronary care package whilst experiencing chest pain, dyspnoea and shock.

The market economy of health care has created an arena in which packages of care can be bought and sold. One dimension of this, for those who wish and can afford it, is the option of buying private health insurance which, they are led to believe, provides a better level of service. Another dimension is that of managed care. This is intended to integrate the activities of health care professionals to achieve a 'patient focused, needs driven, outcomes based approach to care' (Benton 1995). In this context care is matched against a timeline (Fig. 5.2) which specifies the expected timing of critical events. Allied to this critical pathway is a care map which identifies the multidisciplinary team's actions (Hampton 1993).

Discussion

Discussion Topic 5.2

Who co-ordinates care in your practice area?

In what ways could that co-ordination of care be improved?

What should be the nurse's role?

The implications of such packages are enormous. On the positive side they can improve the co-ordination of multidisciplinary treatment and care, increase the demand for research and evidence-based practice, ensure cost containment and facilitate discharge planning (Stahl 1995, Benton 1995, Guanowsky 1995). However, they may also increase both patients' expectations and the risk of litigation if there is deviation from the package (Guanowsky 1995).

At present, in the UK, the sale of packages is confined to local trading between purchasing and providing authorities plus the independent health care sector. With the development of managed care programmes to co-ordinate care for specific client groups, there is no reason why a successful package should not be franchised for use by other authorities on payment of a fee. It is also possible that packages could be advertised for sale directly to potential individual clients through for example Ceefax or the internet

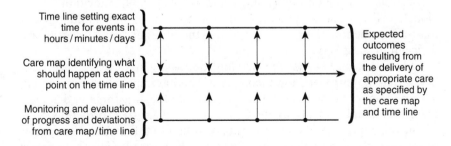

Fig. 5.2 Managed care.

(Benton 1995). The client could be offered a range of income-related packages, which, Stahl (1995) argues, is already happening in North America. Some packages could be based on minimal levels of treatment and care. This raises the question of how far cost cutting can go before the package becomes too cheap to be effective. Similarly, packages could provide excess treatment and care, given solely on the grounds that the client could afford it.

Nurses will have to concern themselves with the business of developing packages of care and identifying potential client markets. The health as a commodity model may not be aesthetically pleasing but it is none the less a reality. It must be considered in any developing framework for care.

THE HEALTH AS AN IDEAL STATE MODEL

The World Health Organization has defined health as 'a state of complete physical, mental and social well-being and not merely the absence of disease and infirmity' (World Health Organization 1946). This model seeks to encompass all aspects of the person which are given equal weighting. It has the added advantage of demonstrating an awareness, through the use of the term 'well-being' that there is more to health than the absence of illness. This, then, is a model with a very broad scope, which seeks to move away from the biotechnological view, towards a more holistic appraisal of health.

Usefulness to nursing

There are several difficulties with this model which make it problematic for use in nursing. To begin with, it is not at all clear what is meant by 'complete physical, mental and social well being' and it is therefore difficult to ascertain how or when these can be achieved. Health, therefore becomes a field with no boundaries whatsoever, in which a person can be described as unhealthy 'if she is unhappy, or bored, or living on her own in a terraced house in Warrington when she wants to be married and living in France' (Seedhouse 1991).

The view of health put forward here, is that of an ideal state which 'sets up a decontextualized standard that ignores personal and social resources, constraints and possibility' (Benner and Wrubel 1989). Inevitably, individuals will feel that they cannot measure up to such high standards and that it is somehow their own fault; that they, rather than the ideal, are deficient in some way.

The model implies that the sick and disabled cannot experience well-being, that they are somehow incomplete. This has implications for nursing in providing services for those with conditions such as asthma or diabetes. Such individuals may be quite well and symptom free, providing they follow the appropriate treatment but according to this model they cannot possess health because they have a disease. There are also implications for those with disabilities, in implying that they also cannot experience well-being. Overall one must conclude that this model is not helpful to nursing.

THE HEALTH AS COPING MODEL

The individual is confronted by life events which challenge the ability to fulfil social roles. Health is therefore a state of optimum capacity which enables the individual to enact roles and carry out tasks. Challenges to the individual's status quo can be large or small. The point is that they are personally significant. To remain healthy the individual must develop coping strategies and adapt to changing circumstances. Failure to achieve this can result in illness which is seen as maladaptive behaviour.

Discussion Topic 5.3

Which model of health is used in your practice area?

What are the strengths and weaknesses of this model in your practice?

Discussion

Usefulness to nursing

This model is widely applied in nursing, for example, by Roy (1984) who regards health as an adaptive state. In her view the individual is a bio-psycho-social being, constantly bombarded by three types of stimuli from the environment:

- Focal – those factors which immediately affect the individual.
- Contextual – those factors occurring alongside the focal stimuli either contributing to them or arising as a result.
- Residual – other factors affecting behaviour for example past experience and values.

The individual has two coping mechanisms. The regulator provides for the physiological dimensions of coping through the neurological and endocrine systems in the body. The cognator system is concerned with cognitive dimensions of coping and effecting change, through thinking and feeling. Change then occurs in one or more of the four adaptive modes. The aim is to achieve harmony and homoeostasis in the individual (Roy 1984).

This concept of health as coping has a widespread applicability in nursing. Health is not seen as a single entity, nor is it related solely to the absence of disease or infirmity. Individuals can be placed at the centre of things, as the yardstick for their own health. Consequently it is possible to have a condition such as hypertension and still be considered healthy if you feel that you are able to cope with and manage your health problems. You are not required to live up to any external notion of health. Health is therefore far more individualistic. Secondly it is subject to change. If, as Roy suggests, the individual is constantly bombarded by stimuli, then s/he is in a constant state of coping and change. Thus, as nurses, we are able to recognize that the individual may be able to manage their hypertension one day but not the next because that hypertension has to be managed alongside a lot of other stimuli.

We can apply this idea of coping in many different ways. For example, it can be used to underpin patient education; helping people to adapt to living with conditions such as asthma or diabetes or altered body image following surgery. It is useful when planning and explaining rehabilitation programmes, in tackling both physiologically and cognitively based problems. Roy's model in particular has been successfully applied in a number of different settings which include caesarian births, care of older persons and those with raised temperatures (Fraser 1996) and found to be valid.

However it is important to recognize that adaptation is to a great extent dependent on motivation and personal resources which not everyone possesses in equal measure, for all sorts of reasons. Each individual does not have the same resilience in coping with illness or with life's problems as everyone else. People do not have the same resources to help them cope. In some instances the presence of illness, such as cancer, may make adaptation virtually impossible and begs the question of whether death is an acceptable form of adaptation or a maladaptive behaviour. This is not as frivolous as it sounds because adaptation takes place within the individual. It is his/her responsibility. Failure to achieve positive adaptation could be used as a form of censure, with the individual being seen as at fault in some way. Secondly there is an implication that the individual who cannot cope is somehow unhealthy. We all have bad days when everything which can conceivably go wrong, does so. If we feel overwhelmed and thus unable to cope, we are, according to this model, unhealthy (Seedhouse 1991).

TOWARDS A POSITIVE MODEL OF HEALTH

There are many different ways of looking at health, most of which appear incompatible with one another and all of which have only limited application in nursing. There is no single definition of health; no single model emerges as entirely helpful. However it is evident that:

- Health is more than the absence of disease.
- It is possible to be healthy but still have illness or disability.
- Ideas about health must reflect equally the experiences of men and women, the racial and ethnic groups to which they belong and the different societies in which they live.
- Health is not static. It is influenced by many factors from both within and outside the individual.
- If health is defined by the individual, then it is not a single state because each person is unique.
- Health as an ideal state is unattainable.

- Individuals cannot take responsibility for every aspect of their health and should not be blamed for this.
- Reductionist models have some usefulness but do not facilitate consideration of the individual's wishes or circumstances.
- Specific models of health are useful to nurses, depending on their client groups, but no one model is universally applicable to all.

A successful theory of health must be based not only on how the individual is now, but what that person might become in both positive and negative terms. It should 'be concerned to identify one or more human potentials which might develop, but which are present or likely to be blocked' (Seedhouse 1991). It 'must be based on an integrated view of mind, body and spirit, and must be based on situated possibility' (Benner and Wrubel 1989). Health work then becomes a process of discovering and, where possible, removing obstacles to human potential. The nature of those obstacles may vary depending on the model of health used. If the model does not allow a focus on those obstacles then it cannot be said to be a theory of health (Seedhouse 1991).

In this context health is based on a phenomenological view of the person, considering the whole person both now and in the future. It allows for illness to be treated and managed but recognizes that the overcoming of disease is not the only priority (Seedhouse 1991). An individual can achieve a state of health whilst still experiencing illness. This challenges the concept of a health–illness continuum. If health is more than the absence of illness; if health and illness can coexist in the same person, then it is possible that the continuum does not exist; that health and illness are separate entities (Seedhouse 1991) with no existence outside the person, except as abstract concepts.

If this is the case then we have to move away from the idea of awarding the patient a score on that continuum. The nurse has to look at the person as a whole; determine the beliefs and meanings which can be ascribed to health and illness and how these coexist within a particular individual. Only then can we begin to make explicit the lived experience of health and illness.

Individuals' beliefs about health are an important factor in nursing assessment. They reflect the individual's underlying value system, their priorities and expectations. Health beliefs reveal the influence of values and beliefs, family, friends, and culture on the individual's understanding of health and illness. These may have little to do with biotechnological explanations. For example health for some Saudi women may be a gift from God (Daly 1995). The factors which influence health beliefs include the behaviours which are considered acceptable and those which are not. Thus if health is solely a gift from God, then only God should be thanked for this. The individual does nothing to merit health and God can take health away perhaps as a punishment or a test. In this situation the individual can do nothing and feels powerless.

Health beliefs therefore reveal the degree of control which individuals feel they have over their health, which will in turn affect their ability to comply with treatment and health education. Those who believe that they can affect their own health are likely to show 'more positive behaviour in taking medication, making and keeping appointments with doctors, maintaining diets and giving up smoking' (McAllister and Farquhar 1992).

It is important for the nurse to be able to recognize and respect each individual's health beliefs. The nurse should take special care not to appear judgmental or critical of people who hold different beliefs. The nurse has an important role to play in ensuring that individuals can access health services on an equal basis (Congress and Lyons 1992). A part of that access lies in humanizing those services; structuring them in a way which accords with the individual's views where this is possible and seeking to work within his/her framework of belief where change has to be effected (Leininger 1985).

WHY IS HEALTH IMPORTANT IN NURSING?

This may seem a rather strange question. Readers of this book are most likely to be health care professionals whose choice of career centred around health issues. We became nurses because we wanted to help and care for people. We saw these activities as important and worthwhile. Nurses who qualified before the introduction of Project 2000, were mostly trained to care for the sick without any consideration of health. As a consequence, our knowledge base was unbalanced, always emphasizing the abnormal without ever allowing us to develop any understanding of what might be considered normal or the social problems with which people had to cope. Thus as a student nurse I felt perfectly confident in caring for children with heart disease but the admission of a normal, abandoned baby utterly confused me.

Discussion

Discussion Topic 5.4

In what ways does a knowledge of health inform and assist your practice?

In recent years nurse education has tried to address this issue. Project 2000 courses were intended to help students develop an understanding of health as well as illness; to develop an appreciation of illness as an event in an otherwise healthy life so that care and treatment can be structured to facilitate a return to that life, in part if not in full. Nursing has invested heavily in health, assigning a high value to it and placing it as a central element in the work of the profession.

In making health a focus for our concern, the concept of a health care professional changes because it has to encompass 'a far wider array of potential and actual colleagues than the traditional hospital or GP-based grouping of doctor, nurse and therapists' (Greenwell 1995). In valuing health we are able to see the person in a more holistic manner by developing an understanding of the individual's lifestyle and circumstances which may contribute to illness or support and care during recovery. We are also able to develop insight into the individual's interpretation and explanation of illness, the consequences of that illness and the actual or potential harm which may arise as a result (Doyal 1995). Such insights enable us to identify the individual's priorities and incorporate these into nursing care. Health is therefore a foundation for holistic care.

The current emphasis on health is to be welcomed but it should not be allowed to obscure illness or the suffering it causes. In examining Project 2000 courses it sometimes seems that the pendulum has swung too far; that today's students are required to concentrate on health in much the same way as previous generations focused solely on illness. The result is that modern students feel as ill-equipped to provide hands on care for the sick, as their predecessors felt about providing health education. It is more than a question of striking a balance between the two because the sick and the dying will always be there; will always need care. Providing this is the proper work of nursing. It should not be delegated to others with less knowledge and skill, nor should it be devalued. Nursing has a responsibility to the sick and the dying which other professions cannot discharge. It also has a duty to ensure that its students are adequately equipped to carry on this work. Nurse theorists must make plain that caring for the sick and dying is a central focus of nursing and not a byproduct.

Exercise 5.1 Developing your own approach to care: health

What do you think health is?

Can you identify any events, people or reading which have influenced your views of health?

Ask a small number of patients in your practice area what they think health is. Are their views different to yours? Can you identify any reasons for these differences?

Record your answers on flip chart material if possible.

Exercises

SUMMARY

This chapter has examined some of the current models of health in terms of their usefulness to nursing. Holistic approaches to health are more helpful because they enable us to place illness within the individual's overall schema and to appreciate that there is more to health than the absence of disease. The individual's health beliefs are an essential part of the nurse's assessment and contribute towards the provision of appropriate individualized care.

Health is a central element in nursing. It enables the nurse to see patients in the wider context of their daily lives and that illness as an event in an otherwise healthy life. However, an overemphasis on health can serve to undermine one of the principal functions of nursing which is caring for the sick and the dying. The profession has a responsibility to prevent this from happening.

REFERENCES

Airhihenbuwa, C.O. (1995) *Health and culture*, Sage, London.

Beattie, A. (1995) War and peace among the health tribes. *In:* Soothill, K., Mackay, L. and Webb, C. (eds) (1995) *Interprofessional relations in health care*, Edward Arnold, London.

Benner, P. and Wrubel, J. (1989) *The primacy of caring: stress and coping in health and illness*, Addison-Wesley, Menlo Park, Calif.

Benton, D. (1995) The role of managed care in overcoming fragmentation. *Nursing Times* 91 (29), 25–28.

Chinn, P. and Kramer, M. (1991) *Theory and nursing: a systematic approach*, Mosby Year Book, St Louis.

Congress, E. and Lyons, B. (1992) Cultural differences in health beliefs: implications for social work practice in health care settings. *Social Work in Health Care* 17 (3), 81–96.

Daly, E. B. (1995) Health meanings of Saudi women. *Journal of Advanced Nursing* 21 May, 853–857.

Doyal, L. (1995) *What makes women sick*, Macmillan, London.

Fawcett, J. (1995) *Analysis and evaluation of conceptual models of nursing*, 3rd edn, FA Davis C, Philadelphia.

Fraser, M. (1996) *Conceptual nursing in practice: a research based approach*, 2nd edn, Chapman and Hall, London.

Greenwell, J. (1995) Patients and professionals. *In*: Soothill, K., Mackay, L. and Webb, C. (eds) *Interprofessional relations in health care*, Edward Arnold, London.

Guanowsky, G. (1995) Liability in managed care for the health care provider. *Nursing Management* 26 (10), 24–25.

Hampton, D. (1993) Implementing a managed care framework through care maps. *JONA* 23 (5), 21–27.

King, I. (1981) *A theory for nursing: systems, concepts, process*, John Wiley and Sons, New York.

Leininger, M. (1985) Transcultural nursing diversity and universality: a theory of nursing. *Nursing and health care* 6 (4), 209–212.

McAllister, G. and Farquhar, M. (1992) Health beliefs a cultural division? *Journal of Advanced Nursing* 17 Dec., 1447–1454.

Naidoo, J. (1986) *Limits to individualism. In*: Rodmell, S. and Watt, A. (eds) *The politics of health education: raising the issues*, Routledge and Kegan Paul, London.

Nightingale, F. (1860/1969) *Notes on nursing*. Dover publications, New York.

Peplau, H. (1952) *Interpersonal relations in nursing*. GP Putnam, New York.

Raymond, N. and D'Eramo-Melkus, G. (1993) Non-insulin-dependent diabetics and obesity in the black and Hispanic population: culturally sensitive management. *Diabetes Education* Jul–Aug, 19 (4), 313–317.

Roper, N. Logan, W. and Tierney, A. (1990) *The elements of nursing*, 3rd edn, Churchill Livingstone, Edinburgh.

Roy, C. (1984) *Introduction to nursing: an adaptation model*, 2nd edn, Prentice Hall, Englewood Cliffs, NJ.

Seedhouse, D. (1991) *Liberating medicine*. John Wiley and Sons, Chichester.

Simpson, H. (1991) *Peplau's model in action*, Macmillan, Basingstoke.

Stahl, D. (1995) Managed care and subacute care: a partnership of choice. *Nursing Management* January, 17–19.

World Health Organization (1946) Constitution, WHO, Geneva.

6 The environment

A COMPARISON OF NURSE THEORISTS' VIEWS OF THE ENVIRONMENT

According to Fawcett (1995) the environment is multidimensional. It incorporates the physical settings in which the individual normally lives, works and socializes. Such settings can have positive or negative effects on a person's health and so need to be considered as part of nursing care. An individual's environment also has psychological and emotional dimensions (Fawcett 1995) which enable the person to interact with others in many different ways: for example, exchanging information, being sociable, teaching and showing affection. These interactions can have an effect on well being and thus affect a person's health. This chapter will help you examine these ideas about the environment in relation to your own field of practice. This will involve looking at some of the ideas put forward by nurse theorists but the main objective is to help you take a fresh look at the pros and cons of the setting in which you work. Figure 6.1 gives an overview of the ideas of nurse theorists to help you begin.

In comparing these theorists' views it is possible to make some statements about the nature of the environment in relation to nursing. First of all it is evident that the concept of these theorists share Fawcett's (1995) view that the environment is complex rather than a single entity. Four of them (King, Roy, Levine, Neuman) see the environment as having an internal dimension, within the person. This comprises both physiological and psychological components which enable the theorists to explore events which occur within the body or the mind. This internal environment is dynamic in that it changes in response to internal events and external stimuli. It can also be a source of stress which challenges the individual and necessitates change.

Discussion

Discussion Topic 6.1

How far is it helpful to think of patients/clients as having an internal environment? What dimensions can you see in this environment?

All the theorists share a view of the environment as external to the person but this can vary between the notion of simply everything outside the body

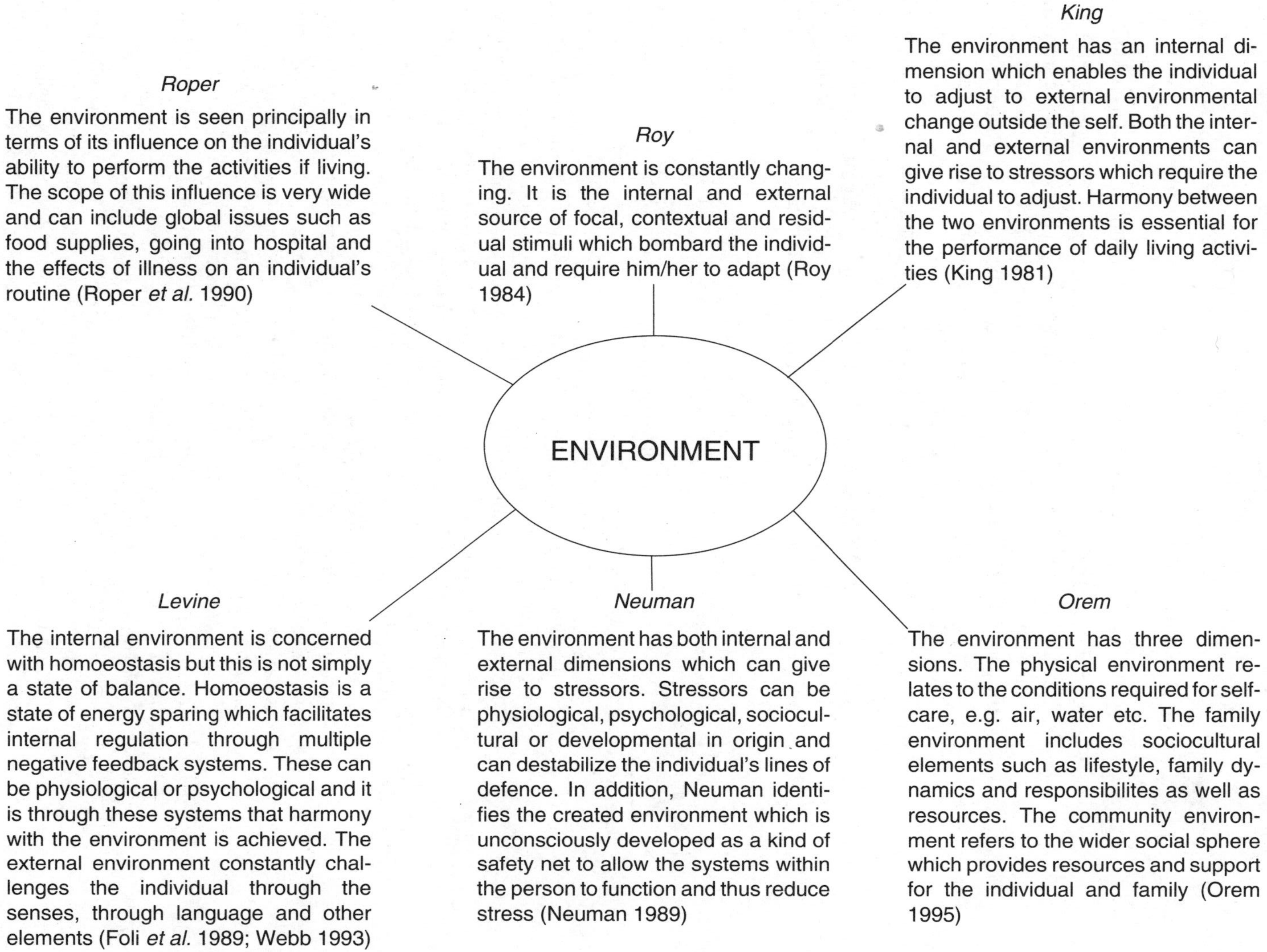

Roper

The environment is seen principally in terms of its influence on the individual's ability to perform the activities if living. The scope of this influence is very wide and can include global issues such as food supplies, going into hospital and the effects of illness on an individual's routine (Roper *et al.* 1990)

Roy

The environment is constantly changing. It is the internal and external source of focal, contextual and residual stimuli which bombard the individual and require him/her to adapt (Roy 1984)

King

The environment has an internal dimension which enables the individual to adjust to external environmental change outside the self. Both the internal and external environments can give rise to stressors which require the individual to adjust. Harmony between the two environments is essential for the performance of daily living activities (King 1981)

Levine

The internal environment is concerned with homoeostasis but this is not simply a state of balance. Homoeostasis is a state of energy sparing which facilitates internal regulation through multiple negative feedback systems. These can be physiological or psychological and it is through these systems that harmony with the environment is achieved. The external environment constantly challenges the individual through the senses, through language and other elements (Foli *et al.* 1989; Webb 1993)

Neuman

The environment has both internal and external dimensions which can give rise to stressors. Stressors can be physiological, psychological, sociocultural or developmental in origin and can destabilize the individual's lines of defence. In addition, Neuman identifies the created environment which is unconsciously developed as a kind of safety net to allow the systems within the person to function and thus reduce stress (Neuman 1989)

Orem

The environment has three dimensions. The physical environment relates to the conditions required for self-care, e.g. air, water etc. The family environment includes sociocultural elements such as lifestyle, family dynamics and responsibilites as well as resources. The community environment refers to the wider social sphere which provides resources and support for the individual and family (Orem 1995)

ENVIRONMENT

Fig. 6.1 An overview of nursing theorists' views of the environment.

(Roper) to that of physical, social and abstract environments which coexist (Neuman, Orem). The external environment can be supportive; providing resources and help (Orem). It can also be challenging, providing stimuli which bring about change in the person (Roy).

> **Discussion Topic 6.2**
>
> How do you see the external environment? What dimensions does it contain?

The environment as a whole is portrayed in an active sense as something which directly affects the person's ability to function, in particular, through the production of stressors or stimuli. In some instances (Roper) the person seems passive; experiencing the effects of changes such as hospitalization. Other theorists see the person as more active. The stressors or stimuli provoke responses from the person who has to adapt in some way in order to maintain some sort of balance, harmony or homoeostasis (Levine, Roy, King, Neuman). In these theories there is an image of interaction between the person and the environment, with each one influencing the other. Thus both are constantly changing because of the demands they make on each other.

> **Exercise 6.3**
>
> Do you see the patient/client as passive, being acted upon by the environment, or capable of affecting it in some way?

Finally Neuman suggests that the person can, in addition to internal and external environments, develop a third dimension which she calls the 'created environment'. This is an abstract environment created by the person, in contrast to the other dimensions which occur naturally. In Neuman's view, the person is composed of several different systems. The created environment helps to integrate these and ensure that they function effectively.

In comparing these different views it is evident that the concepts of the person, health and the environment are closely interlinked. Whilst we might separate them for convenience, we cannot place each of them in isolation. It is impossible to consider the person as being outside of any environment. Even if we disregard the notion of an internal environment we cannot remove the person from the physical environment. The individual may move from one physical environment to another but cannot move out of the environment altogether.

All environments affect health, either in a physical or psychological way or both. Health and the lack of it, can have a profound effect on both the way in which a person is perceived and functions in different environments. Consequently it would seem that the concepts of the person, health and the environment are inextricably linked and that those links are dynamic with each responding to changes in the other two.

Discussion Topic 6.4

What factors in your practice area affect people's health?

This situation can make the environment the most difficult element of nursing to define and may be the reason why the majority of nurse theorists seem to have such difficulty in explaining their ideas. Statements such as 'the created-environment is dynamic and represents the client's unconscious mobilization of all system variables, including the basic structure energy factors, toward system integration stability and integrity' (Neuman 1989) are not helpful and simply serve to fuel antagonism towards theoretical ideas (Miller 1985). The concepts of the person, health and nursing are, by and large, much more clearly set out and seem to have far greater emphasis placed on them.

NIGHTINGALE'S THEORY

To find a nursing theory which both emphasizes the environment and is reader friendly, it is helpful to look at Nightingale (1860/1969). For her the environment is the central focus and she identifies elements within it which affect health. The first is ventilation 'to keep the air he breathes as pure as the external air, without chilling him' (Nightingale 1860/1969). This is 'the first essential to a patient, without which all the rest you can do for him is as nothing' (Nightingale 1860/1969). Unnecessary noise, regardless of its volume, is injurious to the sick. Whispering within earshot of patients, waking them suddenly, hurry and bustle, all disturb the calmness which should prevail in an environment in which the sick are nursed. Cleanliness is also essential. Nightingale writes at some length about the dust that can accumulate on wallpaper or carpets and which will affect the quality of the air in the room. In addition the patient must be washed regularly because 'just as it is necessary to renew the air around a sick person frequently, to carry off morbid effluvia from the lungs and the skin, by maintaining free ventilation, so it is necessary to keep the pores of the skin free from all obstructing excretions. The object both of ventilation and skin cleanliness is pretty much the same – to wit, removing noxious matter from the system as rapidly as possible' (Nightingale 1860/1969). Finally, though by no means the least consideration, is the importance of light, especially sunlight, to both psychological and physical well being.

Nightingale's ideas must be seen within the context of the period in which she was writing. The notion of germs or bacteria which could cause disease was still a radically new concept which Nightingale clearly did not accept. Her ideas about the environment and its effects on health reflect an older concept of disease causation in which it was thought that foul air, amongst other things, could create miasmas. These were thought to be sticky, invisible substances which could adhere to skin and clothing or be inhaled. Direct contact or inhalation could cause disease through the production of humours. There were no covered sewers or waste disposal services. People threw rubbish, including the contents of chamber pots, into the open sewer in the street. It is hardly surprising that, especially in warm weather, the towns and villages stank or that scientific investigation, based solely on observation, concluded that the smell was enough to make people sick (Cipolla 1992).

In her writings, Nightingale shows that she agrees with this. For example a case of pyaemia in a large private house was caused by 'the sewer air (which) was carefully conducted into all the rooms by sedulously opening all the doors, and closing all the passage windows' (Nightingale 1860/1969). In another example she states that 'people have no idea in what good drainage consists. They think that a sewer in the street and a pipe leading to it from the house is good drainage. All the while the sewer maybe nothing but a laboratory from which epidemic disease and ill health is being distilled into the house' (Nightingale 1860/1969).

Knowledge about the spread and control of infection has increased enormously since Nightingale's day and yet the points she raises are still relevant in caring for the sick. Fresh air, light, cleanliness and freedom from unwanted noise are still important in producing a sense of well being, especially amongst those who are very ill or in pain. An additional reason for considering them, is that Nightingale's ideas permeated nurse education in the UK and her influence can be seen in the work of both Henderson (1966) and Roper *et al.* (1990). In developing your own approach to care it can be helpful to identify such influences and decide whether or not they are still applicable to your field of practice

Exercises

> **Exercise 6.1 Developing your own approach to care: the environment**
>
> With reference to your practice area:
>
> - Which aspects of the environment are most important and why?
> - Which aspects of the environment are least important and why?

THE ENVIRONMENT FOR NURSING

A different aspect of the environment is that of the setting in which care is delivered. The settings for nursing care are diverse and include homes, places of work and possibly even some leisure facilities. Practice therefore has to be adapted to suit the needs of the person in these different settings and this can take place in several different ways.

First of all the adaptation of practice can be affected by the physical environment. In a ward setting, the number of beds, the layout and positioning of features like the nurses' station could affect where patients are placed and whether they will need to be relocated elsewhere in the ward as their condition improves. This in turn can affect the allocation of nurses to patients and the ways in which the delivery of care is organized.

Discussion Topic 6.5

How does the physical environment in which you work affect the way you practice nursing?

The organization which employs the nurse will set out certain expectations. In some places of work, for example, the occupational health nurse may be required to provide a treatment service so that staff do not have to take time off work. This nurse may also have to train first aiders to deal with particular types of accidents. In other work settings, the occupational health nurse may have more of an advisory role assisting the company to minimize hazards.

In addition each organization has its own subculture, a term which loosely translates as 'the way we do things around here' (Birnbaum and Somers 1986, Caroselli 1992). On a formal level this means that the organization will set out its own procedures and policies with which staff are expected to comply. On an informal level, organizational subculture affects the ways in which people behave; how they treat each other, their attitudes to work and who has the power to make decisions. The general receptiveness of the organization to change is rooted in its subculture.

At this stage you may find it helpful to look at your own own organization and identify those factors which may have implications for the delivery of nursing care. Please note there are no 'right' answers but as with other exercises you may find it helpful to record your answers on flip chart paper.

Exercise 6.2 Assessing the environment for nursing

With reference to your practice area try to answer the following questions:

1. How do staff perceive each other?
2. What is the relationship between staff and managers?
3. What activities are routine?
4. What is the status of the work you do?
5. What rituals and traditions does the organization have?
6. Which symbols are worn or used?
7. Who are the heroes/heroines in the organization?
8. How receptive is the organization to change?

Exercises

ASSESSING THE ENVIRONMENT FOR NURSING

1. How do staff perceive each other?

In Trust A, staff respect one another's expertise and recognize that each contributes to patient/client care. Staff perceive each other positively as innately good people to have around, irrespective of which profession or discipline they belong to. They value each other's opinion and the work that each one of them performs. Valuing others is reciprocated so that each member of staff feels that he or she is doing something worthwhile. Problems do arise from time to time but these are dealt with through a mixture of regular staff meetings and established but informal channels of co-operation between different staff groups.

In Trust B, the senior medical staff regularly intimidate the nurses both verbally in front of patients and physically by pushing them, standing too close or blocking doorways. Nurses have an antagonistic attitude to the medical staff and use every opportunity to make life difficult for the junior doctors. There are not enough physiotherapists and those in post cannot cope with the number of patients requiring treatment. There are constant complaints about the poor quality of the service and staff turnover in the physiotherapy department is very high. There are no staff meetings in Trust B because the last manager who tried to organize these could not cope with the aggression between the staff members.

These two scenarios represent extremes but, which comes closest to the situation in which you work? Try to identify those factors which make you feel valued and a member of a team and those which do the opposite.

Working as a member of a team is a fundamental part of practice for many nurses. Even those who see themselves as autonomous rely on others for support or to carry out certain activities when they themselves are away. Working as a team is a way of sharing the workload and the stress but it depends on good communication systems. In Trust A, the nurses's handover is regarded by all staff as crucial in ensuring that information is shared. Once a nurse has received a handover report, s/he is expected to know the most up to date information about each patient and to be able to relay this to the appropriate personnel. Nurses expect to be asked for information, particularly in areas where they are responsible for 24-hour care. In Trust B, nurses do not see themselves as central to the information-sharing process. If asked a question, a nurse is likely to say 'I don't know, I've just come on duty' or 'I've been off for 2 days'. Which pattern of behaviour most closely resembles what happens in your situation? What factors contribute to this?

2. What is the relationship between staff and managers?

In Trust A staff are generally respected by those who manage them. Managers consult with staff asking their opinion on matters to do with patient care and professional practice and incorporate the advice of staff into their decision making. Sometimes they are able to follow this advice but both they and the staff know that managers have additional responsibilities. The managers work as a team, taking into account the advice from staff and the needs of the organization as a whole. Consequently no one individual is responsible for either popular or unpopular decisions.

In Trust B the managers meet together every morning at 08.30am to plan the day's strategy. The room in which they meet is on the top floor but has it's own fire escape and a strong lock on the door. The room contains enough coffee and biscuits to last a week. In Trust B the managers are under siege. Their attitude is one of 'let's do it on them (staff, patients anybody) before they do it on us'. Hatred of the managers is about the only thing which unites the staff.

Do you feel that staff in your practice area are respected by the managers and what makes you feel this way?

3. What activities are routine?

In Trust A the normal duties of each member of staff are set out in a job description. These documents clarify the type of work to be done, lines of accountability and areas of responsibility. They also make clear whether the individual should work alone or as part of a team. The daily workload of each member of staff depends on the needs of patients but managers monitor this and try to ensure that individuals are not overworked. In addition, job descriptions are not rigid. Individuals are able to develop their posts in consultation with their managers and in response to perceived needs within the organization.

Trust A also has a number of committees, through which managers and staff members, work together to generate policies and procedures for the organization as a whole. These documents reflect the values of the organization. For example there is a dress code even for staff who do not wear uniform. Lateness is discouraged but managers have a responsibility to find out the reasons for lateness before implementing a punitive policy. Overall there are policies about employment issues, health and safety and most other elements of life within Trust A, plus a range of agreed procedures for clinical matters.

In Trust B the policies and procedures are all in place but they are drawn up solely by the managers. There are no committees to do this work. Consequently staff complain that the procedures are either not practical or not up to date. Actually this is not true because one of the managers has a friend in Trust A and the policies and procedures in each trust are remarkably similar. In Trust B, however, any infringement of the rules, even when based on matters outside the individual's control, is severely punished.

Similarly, Trust B has job descriptions which set out in quite a lot of detail, what each individual is expected to do. Staff follow these rigidly which annoys the managers. They would prefer staff to be more flexible, to allow for overlap between roles which might help to reduce the staffing budget.

Consider your 'normal working day' and the expectations placed on you. These will include the type and amount of work you are expected to complete, whether you are expected to work alone or as part of a team and so on. What, therefore, are you expected to do in the normal course of a day? Try to highlight the values of the organization, what it considers important and why. For example, lateness may be acceptable, tolerated or severely discouraged. How is lateness regarded in your organization and what is done about it? Similarly are there expectations about the way you dress for work, whether or not staff take breaks and where, how people speak to one another and so on? Do people 'get away with' things for no good reason?

4.   What is the status of the work you do?

In Trust A staff see themselves as working together to provide a service to patients. However, there is a recognition that some staff have a front line role in this because they have particular skills. Doctors and nurses are predictably at the forefront in this because of their role in direct patient treatment and care. Thus even within a fairly egalitarian setting some jobs carry higher status than others, but on the whole this does not cause a problem. In addition, certain individual members of staff have carved out roles for themselves which increase their status and that of the work they do. One of these is the receptionist in the Accident and Emergency Department who is extremely skilled at dealing with anxious, traumatized or aggressive people when they arrive in the department. The other staff have come to rely on his judgement. If he says there's going to be trouble, they take notice and act quickly.

In Trust B the surgeons rule the roost. They see themselves as the most important people in the Trust, far more so than the patients. They have pioneered new techniques which have attracted a lot of good publicity for the Trust. No one wants to upset them so they get everything they demand, and they demand a lot. Other medical disciplines take second place. Nursing is tolerated as a necessary but stupid nuisance and the work of the remaining staff is beneath anyone's notice, unless of course they cease to do it. A recent half day stoppage caused havoc even though all departments had been warned about it in advance.

What is the status of nursing within your practice area? Are there individuals in your workplace who have enhanced their personal status and that of their work by developing a specific role? Has this been done with management support?

5.   What rituals and traditions does the organization have?

Rituals have been justifiably criticized as empty actions (Walsh and Ford 1989); but every organization has traditions and rituals which serve important functions in maintaining its character. Rituals are symbolic actions which embody the values and goals of a group of people (Holland 1993) and can be found in a wide range of everyday activities. Thus it is the meaning behind the activity which is important and not the activity itself.

For example, in Trust A, following the handover report in the mornings, ward staff serve breakfast to the patients and then sit down together in the office and drink a cup of tea. One interpretation of this scenario is that the nurses are wasting time. However, managers turn a blind eye to this activity providing it is not abused. They argue that if staff are to work as a team, they must have some opportunity to meet as one. Sitting down together at the start of the shift can provide that much needed chance to meet informally. It can also provide opportunities for story telling: 'Mr Jones came in last night and this is how I coped'. Telling stories can be an important way of learning how to cope with difficult situations or alleviate stress (Shearing and Ericson 1991).

In Trust B the same rituals take place with the addition of a 'guard'. Each morning a member of staff is posted outside the office to watch in case a manager comes into the ward. Should this happen the guard gives a signal to the other members of staff who are adept at hiding the evidence of their tea break. The managers are determined to catch the staff and a game of cat and mouse is played every day, fuelling antagonism between the two groups.

Consider the rituals that are practised in your place of work. Do these function as ways of enhancing working relationships or are they used to undermine them?

A tradition is also a form of symbolic action which is concerned with passing on things to the next generation. At the hospital in which I trained the ward sisters always showed newly qualified staff how to fold their starched linen caps. In a symbolic way this helped to confirm their new status. Are there particular traditions where you work for example when someone qualifies, at Christmas or other important occasions?

6.   Which symbols are worn or used?

Allied to the subject of rituals and tradition is that of symbols. Nurses have dozens of these – uniforms, badges, buckles, caps, keys etc. (Leininger 1978). Some nurses are extremely attached to their symbols almost equating them with being a nurse because they convey power, status or prestige. Alternatively it may be that people simply like dressing up. In both Trust A and B nurses are very keen to retain all their symbols. In Trust B staff are constantly finding new ways to embellish their uniforms. For example they all wear as many badges as possible to advertise their skills. In Trust A nurses have recently negotiated the reintroduction of hats plus a different coloured uniform for each grade of nurse.

What symbols do people feel strongly about in your place of work and what do these symbols convey?

7.   Who are the heroes/heroines in the organization?

Every organization has members who are held up to other staff as good role models. These individuals may be officially regarded by management as shining examples of what is required. For example, in Trust A an enrolled nurse conducted a literature search examining the latest ideas on the prevention of pressure sores. She presented her findings to the managers and the trust was able to reduce the hire of special beds and mattresses, thus saving money. Who are the people in your organization whom managers regard as good role models and why?

On the other hand, these heroes/heroines may be unofficial, inviting admiration for their ability to flout the system in some way or stand up to oppressive management. Unlike the people who 'get away with things,' these individuals are regarded positively sometimes because they have charismatic personalities or because they are thought to be acting in a just way. For example in Trust B a staff nurse who felt she had been intimidated by a consultant, consulted her union which brought a case against the consultant for bullying. In another example in Trust A, a new manager was appointed to a unit which was considered very traditional and old fashioned. Within a year the unit was seen as progressive, a dynamic place to work. Who are the unofficial heroes/heroines where you work? What have they done and why was it considered so important?

8.   How receptive is the organization to change?

Organizational culture has its advantages in that it can help people to work together, to feel secure and that they belong. This is important particularly in professions which rely so much on team effort. Organizational culture enables people to fit in. However it has to be learned. Think back to when you first came to work in this organization. Who told you about 'the way we do things round here'? Depending on the stage of your career it may have been the nursing auxiliary, the health care assistant, a senior student, a staff nurse or someone more senior.

In Trust A new staff receive an induction programme which introduces them to the organization, but in addition each nurse is assigned a mentor. This mentor is based within the same working environment as the new staff member and is therefore on hand as a source of advice and guidance. The mentor's role is to help the new member of staff adapt to new ways of doings things as set out in the organization's policies and procedures and to learn about the informal channels of communication which facilitate daily working life. Students also have a mentor who fulfils a similar function.

In Trust B there is an induction programme with similar aims and objectives but there is no mentorship scheme. Thus staff are left to find things out for themselves. This increases stress and some staff find it difficult to cope unless someone informally decides to be helpful to them. Despite this Trust B has a strong organizational culture which stifles any desire for change. Stasis has set in and new ideas are regarded as a threat (Caroselli 1992).

Answering these questions will have helped you find some of the positive, and perhaps some of the negative points, about the environment in which you work. It may be that you have found more negative than positive factors. After all this is the real world. These strengths and weaknesses can have a profound influence on the way in which you practise nursing. Developing your own approach to nursing must take account of these influences and seek to incorporate at least some of them to ensure successful application of your ideas.

SUMMARY

This chapter has examined the concept of the environment as a central focus for nursing. This is defined in different ways by nurse theorists but in modern terms the individual has an internal and an external environment. The internal environment is composed of physical and psychological elements which interact with each other and with the world outside the person. As a result, the individual both experiences and effects change. Practitioners need to explore the nature of the person's environments and the ways in which these can affect health because these three concepts are inextricably linked.

The environment also includes the setting in which nursing care is given to patients or clients. This can be considered first of all in terms of the geography of the practice area which may affect the ways in which care is organized and delivered. Secondly, health care organizations such as NHS Trusts can create environments for care which reflect their individual values.

Nursing care is delivered within a wide range of environments. It can occur wherever the person happens to be but must be adapted to suit individual needs and the particular setting. This adaptation must also take into account the environment created by the organization which employs the nurse and the occupational subcultures in which individual nurses are required to practise. In developing your own approach to care it is necessary to consider both the environment for care and that of the person. Such consideration creates the foundation of the nurse–patient relationship and allows for diversity in practice.

REFERENCES

Birnbaum, D. and Somers, M. (1986) The influence of occupational image subculture on job attitudes, job performance and job-attitude–job-performance relationship. *Human Relations* 39 (7), 661–672.

Caroselli, C. (1992) Assessment of organizational culture: a tool for professional success. *Orthopaedic nursing* May–June 11 (3), 57–63.

Cipolla, M. (1992) *Miasmas and diseases. Public health and the environment in the pre-industrial age*, Yale University Press, London.

Fawcett, J. (1995) *Analysis and evaluation of conceptual models of nursing*, 3rd edn, F.A. Davis, Philadelphia.

Foli, K., Johnson, T., Marriner-Twomey, A., Poat, C., Poppa, L., Woeste, R. and Zoretich, S. (1989) *Myra Ernestine Levine: four conservation principles. In*: Marriner-Twomey, A. (ed.) *Nursing theorists and their works*, 2nd edn, CV Mosby, St Louis.

Henderson, V. (1966) *The nature of nursing*, Macmillan, New York.

Holland, C. K. (1993) An ethnographic study of nursing culture as an exploration for determining the existence of a system of ritual. *Journal of Advanced Nursing* 18, 1461–1470.

King, I. (1981) *A theory for nursing: systems, concepts, process*, John Wiley and Sons, New York.

Leininger, M. (1978) *Transcultural nursing: theories and concepts*, John Wiley and Sons, New York.

Miller, A. (1985) The relationship between nursing theory and nursing practice. *Journal of Advanced Nursing* 10, 417–424.

Neuman, B. (1989) *The Neuman systems model.* Appleton and Lange, 2nd edn, Norwalk, Connecticut.

Nightingale, F. (1860/1969) *Notes on nursing: what it is and what it is not*, Dover Publications, New York.

Orem, D. (1995) *Nursing, concepts of practice*, 5th edn, CV Mosby, St Louis.

Roper, N., Logan, W. and Tierney, A. (1990) *The elements of nursing*, 3rd edn, Churchill Livingstone, Edinburgh.

Roy, C. (1984) *Introduction to nursing: an adaptation model*, Prentice Hall, Englewood Cliffs, New Jersey.

Shearing, C. and Ericson, R. (1991) Culture as figurative action. *British Journal of Sociology* 42, 481–506.

Walsh, M. and Ford, P. (1989) *Nursing rituals: research and rational action*, Heinemann Nursing, Oxford.

Webb, H. (1993) Holistic care following a palliative Hartman's procedure. *British Journal of Nursing* 2 (2), 128–132.

Nursing 7

NURSING AS A CAREER

According to Fawcett (1995) nursing is the activities carried out by professional nurses in assessing, planning, implementing and evaluating nursing services. These services are delivered to the person, in an environment and in a way which takes account of that individual's lifestyle and circumstances in order to help him/her achieve health. This concept of nursing is extremely broad and the aim of this chapter is to help you examine at least some aspects of it in more detail. A useful place to begin is the reasons why we want to nurse; why we chose nursing as a career and what we think about it now.

Discussion Topic 7.1 Why be a nurse?

Spend a few minutes brainstorming the following questions.

1. Think back to when you applied to train as a nurse. What was it that attracted you to nursing? What did you see yourself doing as a nurse?
2. If you were to be asked the same questions today would you give the same answers and why?
3. How would you describe the nursing that you do?

There are no right answers to these questions.

Discussion

Most potential students are asked why they want to be a nurse, usually with the aim of trying to determine whether the individual has a realistic idea of what being a nurse involves. Answers might include a strong desire to help people, a feeling that nursing is a worthwhile activity and a description of nursing tasks such as washing, feeding and toileting patients. It is most likely that you will have changed some of your opinions about nursing in response to ideas and experiences during or after your training. Important here are the reasons why your ideas have changed and what you think nursing is about now. In particular what is *your* nursing about now and what influences it? These are important questions which are not asked often enough by practitioners because they are so busy keeping services afloat. Yet such questions are an essential prerequisite to determining nursing roles as services grow and change.

NURSING AS CARING

You will probably have included the terms 'nursing care' or 'caring for' in answers to Discussion Topic 7.1 because, in the shorthand of nursing, this is what our work is all about; but what do we mean when we talk about 'care' and 'caring'? Is our care and caring any different to that provided by others? Several chain stores 'care', as do car dealers, parents, teachers and some public figures. Nursing, in this context, would appear to be just another part of the great bandwagon of caring.

A considerable amount of effort has gone into establishing caring as a central element in nursing. According to Leininger (1984) care is 'an essential human need for the full development, health maintenance and survival of human beings in all world cultures'. She goes on to say that

> . . . caring refers to the direct (or indirect) nurturant and skilful activities, processes and decisions related to assisting people in such a manner that reflects behavioural attributes which are empathetic, supportive, compassionate, protective, succorant, educational and others dependent on the needs, problems, values and goals of the individual or group being assisted. (Leininger 1984)

In her view caring is the 'essence of and unifying intellectual and practical dimension of professional nursing' (Leininger 1984) whereas curing is associated with medicine. Caring and curing are complementary but it is possible to provide care without cure.

Reading

> **Reading Suggestion 7.1**
>
> In order to care for others we must also care for each other.
>
> Read Halldorsdottir, S. (1990) The essential structure of a caring and an uncaring encounter with a teacher: the perspective of the nursing student, *In:* Leininger, M. and Watson, J. (eds) *The Caring Imperative in Education*, National League for Nursing, New York.
>
> In what ways can nurses care for and support each other?

This appropriation of caring raises a number of concerns. The polarization of caring and curing – nurses care and doctors cure – implies that nurses have a monopoly on caring which must surely be insulting to our medical colleagues. However, the degree of emphasis placed on caring by other professions may not be the same as in nursing. Kleinman (1988), for example, states that the purpose of medicine is 'both the control of disease process and care for the illness experience'. He argues that medicine has made a lot of progress in the first but neglected the latter. Caring should be at the centre of medical practice with more emphasis on listening to patients and treating them as people.

Caring is based on the principle of altruism, that people other than oneself are important (Benner and Wrubel 1989) and thus establishes a basis for giving help. Caring is not a single entity since the nature of help depends on the situation in which it is required and the manner in which it is given. Caring can involve a lot of hard work both physical and emotional and 'it is not about being nice. It is about being honest, present, authentic, and willing to make choices and decisions, as well as to take risks' (Gray 1994).

Discussion Topic 7.2

Mr Taylor has to ask the nurse for a bottle for the third time. He apologises to the nurse, 'I know you're very busy'.

How often do we keep patients waiting or even forget that they have asked for something?

Discussion

THE COST OF CARING

Valuing other people and providing them with help is therefore not a soft option. To begin with, people invariably want help when it is inconvenient for the helper to provide it. Recipients then feel guilty at taking up the helper's time even when the helper is paid to meet their needs. More importantly, application of the concept of altruism in nursing has tended to focus on the importance of others, the patients, at the expense of the self, the nurse (Benner and Wrubel 1989, Bandman and Bandman 1990). This concept has been interpreted in nursing to mean that the nurse must work tirelessly and selflessly for others. Wisdom, reason and moral priorities have not always been considered (Bandman and Bandman 1990) and the self of the nurse has been ignored (Benner and Wrubel 1989). Concern for others has been seen as taking place at the expense of the self. To focus on the self is selfish and undesirable. The self is therefore placed in a position of competition with concern for others and must suffer as a result. Negating the self, failing to support the self or allow space for personal growth and development will in time create anger and resentment.

Two examples help to illustrate this point. Suppose you want to undertake a particular course or study day about some new aspect of your work. All the arrangements are made: the fee is paid, the off duty arranged. At the last moment you are told you cannot go because of staffing shortages. You reapply to go the next time and the same thing happens. It also happens to your colleagues. When you raise the matter with your manager you are told 'the patients must come first'. How does this make you feel? The first time you might accept the manager's reasons but eventually there will come a day when you cannot give a patient what is required because you don't know what to do. How will you feel then?

In another example, the place in which you work is very busy. You and your colleagues are frequently late getting off duty. The manager refuses to pay overtime but there is no chance of time in lieu. How do you feel about this situation? In the short term you might accept it because you want to do your best for the patients and you cannot just walk away from them. Supposing the situation continues for months or even years. How will you feel then?

In both instances you will probably feel angry and resentful because you care about the patients. You may feel embarrassed because you didn't know what to do for a patient, then angry because you were repeatedly denied the opportunity to learn. You may feel exploited because you have to work overtime regularly and then maybe angry because you are losing your enthusiasm for a job which you used to enjoy. In both examples the self of the nurse is placed second to the needs of patients and when this happens repeatedly the nurse is unable to develop as a human being. The nurse is damaged by this negation of the self and is thus less able to meet the needs of patients.

Nurses are not the only health care professionals to suffer from undue emphasis on valuing someone or something at the expense of the self. Medical practitioners have also been encouraged to see themselves as waging a war against disease. To do this it was seen as necessary to immerse oneself in every aspect of the illness, to 'live with it, smell it, breathe it, be jostled out of your nightly stupor thinking of nothing but illness' (Konner 1993). Caring is not solely about meeting the needs of others. If we ourselves are dehumanized, our usefulness to others diminishes. Several studies (e.g., Goffman 1968, Menzies 1970, Smith 1992) have examined the potentially destructive dimension of caring for others.

Menzies (1970) examined the culture of hospital nursing and argued that it rested on the generation of anxiety. She was extremely critical of the amount of anxiety created by and within nurses themselves, particularly among students who were the major deliverers of hands on care. Most of their working time was spent in close physical contact with suffering and dying people yet they received minimal tuition to help and support them. A number of defence systems evolved to enable nurses to cope with the demands placed on them, for example ritual task performance, constant checking to ensure things were right and avoidance of change. However, in Menzies' view, these served to increase stress. The result was a paranoid-schizoid professional culture and a cumbersome inflexible service (Menzies 1970).

Goffman (1968) examined the total institution of the psychiatric hospital. This governed all aspects of the patients' lives requiring them to live, eat, sleep etc. in close proximity to one another without any choice in the matter. The institution provided for all basic physical needs. Privileges could be earned but only through conforming to the system. Goffman's work is often cited as an example of the destructive power of the hospital particularly in relation to long stay patients, the mentally impaired and those too powerless or vulnerable to protest. What is sometimes overlooked is that the system that socialized patients to conform and that ruled their lives, did exactly the same to staff.

Goffman compared the socialization of patients into the hospital with that undergone by new recruits to the army and an enclosed religious order. The new recruits must be resident, wear uniform, do everything as a group and pass through certain rituals which may involve some degree of humiliation. Until quite recently it was mandatory in many schools of nursing for students to be resident at least for the first part of the course. Uniform had to be worn even in class and nurse tutors undertook uniform inspections to ensure that it was worn 'correctly'. Even as the course progressed and students were allowed to come to class in 'mufti' they still had to have their uniforms available to wear to practical sessions and in case of an emergency.

The hospital provided nurses with a home, food, clothing, companionship as well as a place to work. Deductions were made at source from the nurse's salary to cover the costs of this so that until 1969 nurses received only a small allowance for personal expenses. Nursing folklore abounds with stories of the restrictions placed on nurses in their private lives; for example matron's permission had to be sought if a nurse wished to marry; going out for an evening usually meant getting permission from the sister in charge of the nurses' home.

The message was that a 'good' nurse conformed to this regime. What actually tended to happen was that the group or set of students with whom the nurse began training, became the main focus of support. Friendship and loyalty within the set helped the nurse cope with the very real traumas of nursing the sick and the dying as well as circumvent the oppressive rules of the institution just as Goffman's army recruits would fight for each other rather than the army or a cause.

Smith (1992) applied the concept of emotional labour to nursing. This she defines as 'the induction or suppression of feeling to sustain an outward appearance that produces in others a sense of being cared for in a convivial safe place' (Smith 1992). The achievement of this requires considerable effort, education and organizational support since 'caring does not come naturally. Nurses have to work emotionally on themselves in order to appear to care'. The personal dimension of nursing (Carper 1978) is thus essential. Personal growth and development must take place if the nurse is to be able to act as a therapeutic agent (Peplau 1952). Caring in this context is utterly intangible. There is no list of procedures to be applied or equipment to be used. It cannot be itemized and costed and is consequently of little value to those whose job it is to balance the accounts. Smith (1992) is critical of nursing leaders who have exhorted the profession to adopt the concept of caring whilst failing to appreciate or address these issues.

Caring is therefore a complex and potentially dangerous activity. If it is to be placed at the heart of what we do, as virtually synonymous with nursing then we must be clear about two things. First of all we must clarify what we mean by caring and the ways in which nurses' caring differs from that of others. Leininger's (1984) work has made some progress with this but we need to examine caring in relation to our own everyday practice and ask ourselves 'what are the unique elements here that only nurses can provide and why?' Secondly we must be clear about the potential costs of caring for ourselves and our colleagues and consider ways in which these can be minimized.

PROFESSIONAL IMAGES OF NURSING

Many other people – parents, neighbours, those looking after elderly relatives – undertake some of the work which nurses do and consequently there has developed an opinion that anyone can nurse. This is coupled with a popular notion that nursing is a suitable occupation for those who are not academically inclined. During every summer I spent as a senior tutor (in the late 1980s) a number of parents would bring their daughters to my office saying 'She's failed her A-levels. We thought she could do a spot of nursing'.

It has to be acknowledged that nurses contribute to these images of nursing. The average nurse when asked about his/her work will shrug and reply 'I'm just a staff nurse' or 'we just look after them when they come back from theatre'. The implication is that nursing is of very little importance. Never will the nurse reply 'I worked hard for three years to obtain my registration. I had to do additional qualifications in ENT nursing. I am responsible for patients returning from theatre which means I monitor their breathing, blood pressure, pulse and wound for signs of bleeding etc. I also supervise and teach less experienced staff. I deputise for the manager in her absence which means that I am then responsible for the entire ward'.

Look back at the way you described your nursing at the beginning of this chapter. Which type of answer did you give? Was it a dismissive, 'nothing really' sort of answer or did you take the time to set down clearly what you do and what you are responsible for? This is an important step in making nursing explicit. First of all it conveys how we feel about our work and indeed about ourselves. If we lack self-respect, if we are not proud of what we do or are unable to explain clearly our work, it is hardly likely that anyone else will either value or have confidence in it. One of the intentions of the professional portfolio (UKCC 1994) is to help nurses develop a detailed record of experience and learning, to demonstrate ongoing career development. Profiles which reflect the 'I'm just a staff nurse' attitude are not going to be much use in obtaining either academic accreditation or promotion. Finally, the internal market of the NHS requires us to sell our nursing services to purchasers. No one is going to pay for a service which is not clearly and properly defined. If we want to be taken seriously as professionals, equal to other professions, then we must start talking about our work in a more positive manner.

LAY AND PROFESSIONAL NURSING

Leininger (1981) is one of the very few nurse theorists to have addressed the interface between lay and professional nursing. She argues that every society has informal or lay systems to provide care. These systems are locally based, informal and closely intertwined with, for example, social structures, kinship, culture and religion. They rely on low cost, non-technological approaches to care. They offer explanations of health and illness which may have little to do with science. In contrast, the professional

Table 7.1 Lay and professional care

Lay system	Professional system
Tends to be holistic in focus	Tends to be scientific and fragmented in focus
Emphasizes care, non-technological approaches	Emphasizes cure and technological approaches
Low cost	High cost
Uses what is familiar to patients including local resources and home setting	May be quite alien to patients and rely on professional services and maybe hospitals
Emphasis is on group or family	Emphasis is on individual patient
Uses diverse and possibly non-technical explanations of illness and health	Uses scientific explanations of illness and health

(Adapted from Leininger 1981)

health care system is based on formal education based largely on Western ideologies of health and illness. These two systems are very different in their 'philosophy, socialization and role performance' and conflicts may arise between the two (Table 7.1). In order to minimize conflict between the two systems we need to be aware of the differences between them and to relate them to our own care settings. In doing so we have to make clear how we, as professionals, see the nursing we provide; the preferences of our client groups and how we plan to meet their specific nursing needs.

Theorists such as Orem (1995) see the patient as an individual motivated towards self-care and the family as the primary caregivers when the person is unable to meet his/her needs. She argues that the professional nurse intervenes only when the family cannot cope. The nature of that intervention can have three different forms, all of which are intended to facilitate self-care whenever possible. The first level of intervention is 'supportive-educative' in which the nurse provides specific teaching to the patient or family or adopts a counselling role to assist people to resolve problems. In some instances this type of intervention may be all that is required. Some patients will need additional help or 'partly compensatory' intervention in which the nurse performs certain tasks which the patient is unable or unwilling to do so. Others will be totally dependent on the nurse and require 'wholly compensatory' intervention. However even at this stage it may be possible to encourage some small act of independence. Orem therefore sees nursing in terms of clearly defined actions to achieve specific aims whilst working within the framework of the patient's preference for self-care.

In contrast Leininger (Leininger 1985) sees the patient as wanting culturally appropriate nursing care. She also outlines three types of intervention available to the nurse. Cultural care preservation strategies allow the nurse to work within the patient's culture; for example, in providing health education. Cultural care accommodation interventions are intended to help the patient adapt to changes such as the management of diabetes in a culturally acceptable way. Cultural care repatterning strategies help the patient cope with major changes in life – following the formation of a stoma, for example.

It is acknowledged that these examples are very broad but the principle is that nurses should be able to identify the nursing needs and preferences of local populations. This is an essential part of the mixed economy of care introduced by recent health service reform which requires more efficient use of public monies through assessment of client needs; prioritizing needs and tailoring services to meet them (White Paper 1989, Meredith 1993).

THE NURSING PROCESS

The nursing process developed alongside movements to provide more holistic and individualized nursing care together with a rational base for nursing action. The achievement of these elements was regarded as an important prerequisite to independent professional status. The process is essentially a decision making pathway (Kratz 1979),

> . . . an orderly, systematic manner of determining the client's health status, specifying problems defined as alteration in human need fulfilment, making plans to solve them, initiating and implementing the plan, evaluating the extent to which the plan was effective in promoting optimum wellness and resolving the problems identified. (Yura and Walsh 1988)

This decision making pathway (Fig. 7.1) is dependent upon interaction between the nurse and patient. Whilst it is usually presented as a series of steps, it is in practice a dynamic framework. The first stage is assessment

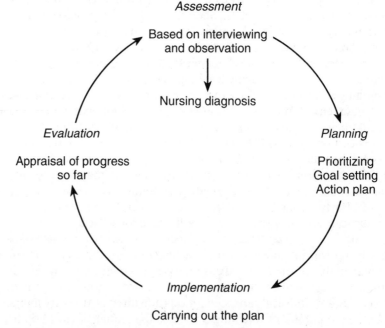

Fig. 7.1 The nursing process.

(Fig. 7.1) which is dependent on two major nursing skills – interviewing and observation. The nurse interviews the patient to obtain information about factors such as lifestyle, social background plus knowledge and views about his/her state of health and how this may have changed. The nurse observes the patient's body language for indicators of his/her mental state and physical signs such as breathing, the condition of the skin and the degree of mobility. The nurse also takes measurements when necessary; for example recording blood pressure or conducting urinalysis.

Discussion

Discussion Topic 7.3 Nursing in your field of practice

What theory is currently used to underpin the nursing process in your practice area and why?

Is this theory used:

- nominally, i.e. just the basic ideas;
- partially, i.e. selected parts of it are used;
- completely, i.e. as the theorist intended?

The nurse superimposes a theory on the decision making pathway for the collection and synthesis of this information. This provides a framework which will determine how the assessment is conducted. For example assessment based on Roper *et al.*'s (1990) theory of nursing will centre on the activities of living with questions related to each activity and the factors which, according to Roper *et al.*, influence it. Assessment based on Roy's (1984) theory would be formulated around the four modes. Each assessment would yield the same information but there might be some differences in emphasis.

Regardless of the framework used, the end product should be the identification of the patient's problems and the formulation of a nursing diagnosis (Fig. 7.1). This is 'a clinical judgement about an individual, family or community which is derived through a deliberate, systematic process of data collection and analysis' (Shoemaker 1985) which provides the rationale for nursing actions. It is essentially a nursing judgement about matters which are within the scope of nursing practice and which can be dealt with by the nurse (Shoemaker 1985). Nursing diagnosis is a complex undertaking in which the practitioner considers a number of issues in relation to the information collected during assessment. These can include the nurse's experience (Watson 1994), the situation of the patient and whether there is a need for medical intervention (Edwards 1994).

Reading

Reading Suggestion 7.2

Read Shoemaker, J. (1985) Characteristics of a nursing diagnosis. *Occupational Health Nursing* August, 387–389.

What is a nursing diagnosis? Look up references to the North American Nursing Diagnosis Association on CD-ROM.

The planning stage (Fig. 7.1) involves using knowledge gained during the assessment to establish priorities. Some theories allow the nurse to undertake this stage alone. For example Nightingale (1860/1969) sees the patient as essentially passive and in certain settings, such as intensive care, such a view may be appropriate. Other theories, for example Peplau (1952), require a partnership with the patient so that the priorities established are negotiated by both parties and not determined solely by the nurse. The establishment of priorities facilitates the setting of goals and the selection of appropriate nursing interventions. It also helps to maintain a strong focus on individualized nursing. Even though some patients may have very similar problems, their priorities and goals will be different.

Goals have to be achievable and realistic. If they are not the patient will become discouraged and maybe cease to trust those providing care. The nurse too will feel frustrated and be unable to demonstrate what has been achieved in the evaluation stage. It is therefore important to devise goals in a way that allows for achievement or otherwise to be clearly documented. A goal should specify:

Who:	Mr Jones
Will do what:	will walk to the toilet twice a day
Using what means:	accompanied by one nurse
To what degree of success:	without stopping to rest
By which date:	by April 29.

This method of constructing goals is mechanistic and has limitations but it does set out clearly what is to be achieved. It also facilitates the construction of individual action plans as no two individuals will have to achieve exactly the same goal. Action plans set out the nursing interventions required to enable the patient to achieve each goal.

These factors form the basis for implementation and evaluation. The action plan is not a rigid formula. The components of the goal allow the patient partial success if the entire goal proves to be too much. They also allow the nurse to identify which aspects of the goal require further intervention. Thus the nurse is constantly evaluating whether or not the patient is able to achieve a particular goal and adjusting either the action plan or even the goals themselves.

The nursing process has been in use in British nursing for over fifteen years. It has been taught to every nurse who has studied for registration during that time plus those undertaking post qualifying courses. The results have been of limited success with many nurses not understanding which theory, if any, they are using to implement the process. Part of the problem was that the process was introduced before nurses had received any education in which they were made aware of theory or any encouragement in identifying the theories they used. Fifteen years of imposing published models of nursing have not helped. It may be that nurses have an inbuilt resistance to such impositions. It is also possible that nurses were not encouraged to gain any deep understanding of the theories involved. The most commonly imposed theory was that by Roper, Logan and Tierney (1990). It would be interesting to know how many nurses actually read their books and can identify the different elements of their theory. It would also be interesting to find out how many nurses use a modified version of Roper *et al.*'s work and how many use the theory correctly. Nurses need to clarify which theories they are actually using as part of achieving credible decisions.

Reading

Reading Suggestion 7.3

Read Mitchell, J. (1984) Is the nursing any business of doctors? A simple guide to the 'nursing process'. *The British Medical Journal* 288, 21 Jan., 216–219.

and

Tierney, A. (1984) A response to Professor Mitchell's simple guide to the nursing process. *British Medical Journal* 288, 17 March, 835–838.

What arguments are put for and against the nursing process and how valid are these now?

THE MEDICAL MODEL

In examining the concept of nursing as 'the actions taken by nurses on behalf of or in conjunction with the person' (Fawcett 1995) we begin to expose some of the weaknesses in Fawcett's ideas. To begin with, the nurse as a person is ignored. It would be easy to say that the nurse can be categorized as a person but that is not enough. The nurse is a particular kind of person with a personality, beliefs, values, motivation, knowledge, skills and attitudes. The nurse has to develop professionally and personally in order to become a therapeutic agent and therefore needs to be considered as separate to the concept of the person as a recipient of nursing care. To categorize the nurse within the dimension of nursing is also unsatisfactory since it denies the humanity of nurses. This omission of the nurse means that nursing theorists do not always consider it either (Taylor 1992) and nurses can therefore be depersonalized in theory just as they are in nursing work.

An additional consideration is the relationship between nursing and other professions. Nursing has to take account of the work of other professionals yet there is nothing in Fawcett's ideas to encourage the practitioner to do so. It is almost as if nursing exists in a vacuum with no one else involved and, as we have seen with the issue of caring, there is sometimes an implied criticism of other professionals. The relationship between nursing and medicine illustrates this point. Nursing theory is portrayed as holistic and patient-centred in implied criticism of the so-called 'medical model'.

What I think nurses mean by this term is the approach by which doctors examine, diagnose and treat patients (Fig. 7.2). This approach is regarded as systematic and scientific. It is widely accepted by doctors as the way to practise and it works sufficiently often to be considered worthwhile. In the

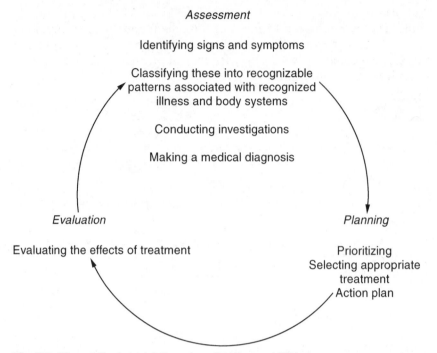

Fig. 7.2 The medical model (based on Seedhouse 1991).

first stage the doctor collects information through physical examination, interviewing the patients about the nature of the problem and conducting a range of tests. This information is then collated and synthesized to form the basis of a medical diagnosis. Further decisions about treatment can then be made and ultimately be evaluated. Superimposed on this 'medical model' is the doctor's knowledge of disease and its manifestations, differential diagnoses and different treatment regimes. Also superimposed is the doctor's framework for practising medicine.

Thus the so-called 'medical model' is not a model at all in the sense that nurses use this word. It is actually a decision making pathway very similar to the nursing process; a medical process (Table 7.2). It facilitates complex decision making in an inexact discipline. Every step of this medical process is filled with uncertainty. The cause of many conditions such as rheumatoid arthritis, coeliac disease, multiple sclerosis and anorexia nervosa are either unknown or uncertain and consequently there may not be clear diagnostic criteria. Even where diagnosis can be achieved there may be a range of possibilities from which to choose (Seedhouse 1991). Chest pain for example could signify a myocardial infarction, angina, or indigestion. The difficulties do not end with diagnosis because the doctor may be confronted by a range of possible treatments most of which have not been evaluated in any systematic way because 'there is no procedure for formally scrutinizing operations or diagnostic tests unless they involve the use of new substances' (Konner 1993). At every stage there is the prospect of making the wrong decision (Seedhouse 1991).

Reading Suggestion 7.4

Read Hunsberger, M., Mitchell, A., Blatz, S., Paes, B., Pinelli, J., Southwell, D., French, S. and Soluk, R. (1992) Definition of an advanced nursing practice role in the NICU: the clinical nurse specialist/neonatal practitioner. *Clinical Nurse Specialist* 6 (2), 91–96.

In what ways do nursing and medical roles overlap in this article? How do roles overlap in your practice area? In what ways should the overlap be acknowledged and what are the implications for practice and care?

Reading

The 'medical model' and the nursing process provide professionals with some sort of basis for decision making. As such they are neutral. Criticisms of the one as reductionist or the other as unrealistic are not appropriate. It is the ways in which each is utilized by individual practitioners which makes the difference between humane, patient centred practice and dehumanized service provision.

Table 7.2 The medical model and the nursing process

Medical	Nursing
Identifying signs and symptoms by interviewing and physical examination	Collecting information by interviewing and observation plus measurement of factors such as blood pressure
Assessment	
Classifying these into recognizable patterns associated with recognized illness and body systems Conducting investigations Making a medical diagnosis	Synthesizing information to identify problem areas Making a nursing diagnosis
Planning	
Prioritizing Selecting appropriate treatment Action plan	Prioritizing Goal setting Action plan
Implementation	
Carrying out the plan	
Evaluation	
Reappraising the effects of treatment	Reappraising the patient's ability to achieve goals and the effects of nursing interventions

THE DOCTOR–NURSE GAME

There is a considerable amount of writing about the working relationships between doctors and nurses (Sweet and Norman 1995) much of which is based on the study of gender-based social roles. Stein (1967) found that nurse–doctor relationships were influenced by these roles and gender based divisions of labour, patriarchy and what she calls the 'doctor–nurse game'. In Stein's analysis doctors were expected always to make correct decisions and were consequently frightened of making mistakes. As a defence mechanism doctors adopted a belief in their own omnipotence. Nurses were socialized to bolster this belief through their subservience. The game consisted of the nurse giving advice to the doctor whilst not appearing to do so. Thus the nurse might say 'the patient appears to have a raised temperature' or even 'the patient appears to have died'. In a follow up to this research, Stein *et al.* (1990) found that the game had changed. A more even distribution of men and women in both medicine and nursing, changing social roles and values and better education for nurses meant that nurses could now give more straightforward advice to doctors.

The development of specialist and advanced nursing roles (UKCC 1994) and the impact of reduction in the junior doctors hours are likely to have considerable impact on the work of both doctors and nurses. It is possible for nurses to be more expert than doctors in particular areas of practice and, in some situations, better educated than their medical colleagues. The old style of working in which the doctor held all the decision making power is no longer appropriate. Both professions have to consider how best to foster the collaborative working relationships which must exist for the benefit of patients (McGee *et al.* 1996).

There is more at stake than interprofessional rivalry. The provision of health care is now a complex business and more dependent than ever on multidisciplinary working. A small survey of nurses and podiatrists (McGee and Ashford 1996) highlighted the need for professionals to have a thorough understanding of each other's roles in order to clarify what each can provide in terms of patient care. A failure to achieve this could mean that patients miss out on essential services because practitioners do not know who provides them.

Discussion

Discussion Topic 7.4 Relationships with other professionals
In your field of practice, which professions interface most regularly with nursing?
Looking at Stein's ideas, how would you describe the relationship between nursing and each of these professions?
What, in detail, does each of these professions contribute to multidisciplinary client/patient care?

SUMMARY

This chapter has examined some of the concepts within nursing. Nursing is about providing care, for example as defined by Leininger (1984) but caring has costs. The nurse can suffer as a result of providing care for others and nursing theory is weak on recognising that nurses are persons with particular needs.

Nursing is seen as a professional activity and differentiated from lay forms of caring. A part of this differentiation must involve raising the self-image and self-respect of nurses who must be able to give a positive account of their contribution to health care.

The nursing process is a decision making framework onto which theoretical ideas can be imposed. It can be compared with the so-called medical model which is another decision making framework with many similarities. Used properly both can provide a basis for systematic care.

Medicine and nursing are undergoing change and the interface between the two needs to be clarified. The old gender based games outlined by Stein (1967) are no longer appropriate. Health care is now a complex business. All professionals need to be fully informed about the role of other members of the multidiciplinary team.

In developing your own approach to nursing there are a number of issues which need to be examined. Nursing is not simply a description of what we do but of how we regard our work, whether we meet the expectations of our patients and the ways in which nursing interrelates with other professional groups. These are complex issues which need time and thought and completing the exercises in this chapter has probably taken you longer than anticipated. You will need all this material for the next chapter which aims to show you how you can use your ideas to develop your own approach to nursing.

REFERENCES

Bandman, E. and Bandman, B. (1990) *Nursing ethics through the lifespan*, Prentice Hall International Edition, London.

Benner, P. and Wrubel, J. (1989) *The primacy of caring: stress and coping in health and illness*, Addison Wesley, Menlo Park, Calif.

Carper, B. (1978) Fundamental patterns of knowing in nursing. *Advances in Nursing Science* 1 (1), 13–23.

Edwards, B. (1994) Telephone triage: how experienced nurses reach decisions. *Journal of Advanced Nursing* 19, 717–724.

Fawcett, J. (1995) *Analysis and evaluation of conceptual models of nursing*, 3rd edn, FA Davis, Philadelphia.

Goffman, E. (1968) *Asylums*, Penguin, Harmondsworth.

Gray, D. P. (1994) *Feminism and nursing, In:* Strickland, O. and Fishman, D. (ed.) *Nursing issues in the 1990s*, Delmar Publishers, New York.

Kleinman, A. (1988) *The illness narratives*, Basic Books, New York.

Konner, M. (1993) *The trouble with medicine*, BBC Books, London.

Kratz, C. (1979) (ed.) *The nursing process*, Baillière Tindall, London.

Leininger, M. (1978) *Transcultural nursing: concepts and theories*, John Wiley and Sons, New York.

Leininger, M. (1981) Transcultural nursing: its progress and its future. *Nursing and Health Care* 2 (7), 365–371.

Leininger, M. (ed.) (1984) *Care, the essence of nursing and health*, Wayne State University Press, Detroit.

Leininger, M. (1985) Transcultural nursing diversity and universality: a theory of nursing. *Nursing and Health Care* 6 (4), 202–212.

McGee, P. and Ashford, R. (1996) Nurses' perceptions of roles in multidisciplinary teams. *Nursing Standard* 10 (45), 34–36.

McGee, P., Castledine, G. and Brown, R. (1996) A survey of specialist and advanced nursing practice in England. *British Journal of Specialist Practice* 2 (2), 682–686.

Menzies, I. (1970) *The functioning of social systems as a defence against anxiety*, Tavistock Institute of Human Relations, London.

Meredith, B. (1993) *The community care handbook: the new system explained*, Age Concern and Ace Books, London.

Nightingale, F. (1860/1969) *Notes on nursing: what it is and what it is not*, Dover Publications, New York.

Orem, D. (1995) *Nursing, concepts of practice*, 5th edn, CV Mosby, St Louis.

Peplau, H. (1952) *Interpersonal relations in nursing*, GP Putnam, New York.

Roper, N., Logan, W. and Tierney, A. (1990) *The elements of nursing*, 3rd edn, Churchill Livingstone, Edinburgh.

Roy, C. (1984) *Introduction to nursing: an adaptation model*, 2nd edn, Prentice Hall, Englewood Cliffs, New Jersey.

Seedhouse, D. (1991) *Liberating medicine*, John Wiley and Sons, Chichester.

Shoemaker, J. (1985) Characteristics of a nursing diagnosis. *Occupational Health Nursing*, August, 387–389.

Smith, P. (1992) *The emotional labour of nursing*, Macmillan, London.

Stein, L. (1967) The doctor–nurse game. *Archives of General Psychiatry* 3 (27), 993–995.

Stein, L., Watts, D. and Howell, T. (1990) The doctor–nurse game revisited. *New England Journal of Medicine* 322 (8), 546–549.

Sweet, S. and Norman, I. (1995) The doctor–nurse relationship: a selective literature review. *Journal of Advanced Nursing* 22, 165–170.

Taylor, B. J. (1992) From helper to human: a reconceptualisation of the nurse as a person. *Journal of Advanced Nursing* 17, 1042–1049.

United Kingdom Central Council for Nursing, Midwifery and Health Visiting (1994) *The future of professional practice – the Council's standards for education and practice following registration*, UKCC, London.

Watson, S. (1994) An exploratory study into a methodology for the examination of decision making by nurses in the clinical area. *Journal of Advanced Nursing* 20, 351–360.

Yura, H. and Walsh, M. (1988) *The nursing process*, 5th edn, Appleton and Lange, Norwalk, Connecticut.

Working for patients (1989) Cm 555, HMSO, London (White paper).

Implementing your own approach to nursing

COLLATING YOUR IDEAS ABOUT NURSING

The last four chapters have examined each of the four elements of Fawcett's (1995) explanation of nursing. In particular these chapters have considered the differing interpretations put forward by nurse theorists and some of the issues which need to be considered in relation to these. As a result we can see that there are quite a number of nurse theorists and that they have produced a range of theories. Most of these can be categorized as developmental, systems-based or interactional (Table 3.1, p. 23). Thus Fawcett's (1995) ideas would appear to be sufficiently neutral to allow for different interpretations but it is clearly not completely so because the range of categories of theory is not very wide. A second criticism is that her explanation ignores the nurse as an individual with particular attributes and needs. It is therefore continuing a trend in nursing in which nurses have been dehumanized. On the whole, nursing theories do not challenge this idea.

Despite these weaknesses Fawcett's work is still very useful in helping us to examine nursing. It also highlights the fact that there is no one nursing theory to which all practitioners must subscribe. Individual interpretation is permissible, even desirable, because in each work setting there are so many variables to consider in terms of the clients, environment, health issues and nursing services. Published theories do not always give what is needed in specific settings and it is therefore important that practitioners identify what they need for their workplace. The first aim of this chapter is to help you begin to do this by collating the material from the exercises throughout the book and identifying factors which have influenced you.

Reading Suggestion 8.1

Read Marriner-Twomey, A. (ed.) (1989) *Nursing theorists and their work*, CV Mosby, St Louis.

Choose any two chapters on individual nurse theorists. What influences can you identify in relation to each theorist? Can you trace any of these influences in the theory?

Reading

Sources of influence can be many and varied. They could include, for example, a particular ward sister or charge nurse who acted as a role model in some way. Throughout my career I have been very conscious of this type of practitioner and had the good fortune to work with some of them. In my experience they have been extremely knowledgeable about their field and experts in their practice. They also possess the ability to pass on, not only their knowledge but their enthusiasm for their subject (McGee 1992).

Patients can also be a considerable source of influence on our developing ideas. Strategies such as total patient care provide opportunities for nurses and patients to get to know one another as human beings. In some instances the nurse gains a privileged insight into the patient's world. This helps to shape our future interactions with others who need our care.

Finally, sources of influence can include books and articles, films, TV and other media. Whilst many of these will be about nursing or nursing-related subjects, others may be from completely outside the field. Ideas do not come solely from within our own professional field. Looking elsewhere can give a new perspective on old ideas. This chapter asks you to identify factors which have influenced your development as a nurse and why.

Exercises

Exercise 8.1 Developing your own approach to care: collating your ideas

You will need to gather together the answers you developed in relation to the following exercises:

- *Person*   Exercise 4.1: The nature of the person.
                    Discussion Topic 4.1 How do you see the person?
                    Exercise 4.3: Developing your own approach to care: the person.
- *Health*   Exercise 5.1: Developing your own approach to care: health.
- *Environment*   Exercise 6.1: Developing your own approach to care: environment.
- *Nursing*   Discussion Topic 7.3: Nursing in your field of practice.

If you have recorded your answers on flip chart material it can be helpful to hang all the pages on the wall. This enables you to see a more complete picture of your ideas and maybe even show them to others if you wish to do so. It also gives you space in which to add extra points.

Take as much time as you wish to answer the following questions.

1. What are the characteristics of the patients or clients for whom I provide a service?
2. Why do I see them in this way? Is it experience alone or have I been influenced by any particular events, people or theory either from nursing or another discipline?
3. Which model of health am I using and why? What has influenced my choice?
4. In which environment(s) do I meet with my patients or clients? What are the characteristics of these environments and how do these affect nursing activities?

5. What is nursing about in my place of work, i.e. what does the work involve?
6. What are the main influences on my nursing activities? Are they people, theories, experiences?

In completing this exercise you will be beginning to clarify your own ideas and identify those you have borrowed from elsewhere. When you have answered these questions try to write a summary of your thoughts about the person, the environment, health and nursing. Set out below are some examples of what your approach might look like.

APPROACH TO NURSING IN A REHABILITATION SETTING

I began to develop this approach to nursing whilst working in a rehabilitation unit which catered mainly for adults who had experienced cerebrovascular accidents. This was the first time I had considered my approach to nursing.

Person

An adult individual with physical and possibly cognitive impairment who has experienced a profound loss of independence. This loss may be physical but may also take other forms. For example the individual may have suffered cognitive rather than physical changes or may have become institutionalized through prolonged hospital stay and dependence on professional care. Independence can also be eroded by the disruption of normal roles as a family member or worker.

Environment

The physical environment exists within the body and in this instance is impaired. This affects everyday activities such as walking. Consequently the physical environment outside the body is unsuitable for the individual who cannot function independently on a physical level without danger to him/herself. The psychological environment includes the person's mental state, cognitive abilities and personality which contribute to the individual's interpretation of internal and external events. In this instance the psychological environment is also impaired and consequently the individual may not be able to think clearly, recognize objects or speak coherently. The ability to interact with the environment outside the self is therefore seriously affected. The social environment consists of the person's family members, and friends as well as work and leisure activities. All of these relationships and activities have been disrupted and are in some need of repair.

Nursing

Nursing is a set of interpersonal and physical skills aimed at enabling the individual to regain and maintain dignity and self-esteem through the facilitation of some degree of independence. Implicit in this type of nursing is a range of subskills including creativity, honesty, manual dexterity, physical strength, patience and management. In the context of nursing patients with multiple disabilities, the overall aim is to create a home, an environment in which individuals can feel sufficiently secure to regain confidence and at least some skills.

Health

Health is a varying state in which the patient is able to maintain family and social relationships; achieve some degree of independence from others in the performance of personal care activities; there is co-ordinated support which minimizes rather than exaggerates dependence.

Sources/influences

Most of the ideas came from experience in nursing patients who had strokes and the insight gained into the nature of their disabilities. A particular influence was a man called Albert who had suffered his third stroke before being admitted to the unit. He was also a diabetic and had hypertension. His previous strokes had left him partially disabled and with limited speech. The first challenge, therefore, was to determine what could realistically be achieved. The nursing staff discussed with Albert and his wife what they felt they could offer; continence training, feeding skills, dressing skills. It quickly became clear that this was not what they wanted. After each of the previous strokes, Albert's wife had found it much quicker to wash and dress him herself, every morning, at the same time as getting the children ready for school. She then went to work and Albert was left on his own in the house until about 1.30 pm. The couple had two priorities as far as rehabilitation was concerned. Albert had to be safe to be left on his own so that his wife could keep her job. He also had to be able to perform a list of jobs which marked his, albeit limited, contribution to the household. These tasks were tidying the sitting room and washing the breakfast dishes plus making a cup of tea and a sandwich for his wife when she came home from work. As far as Albert and his wife were concerned, if he washed and dressed himself he would be too tired to complete his work.

Albert and his wife had a profound influence on my thinking about the nature and purpose of rehabilitation work. In particular, the experience of working with them helped me to listen more clearly to what patients really wanted rather than provide a standard package of care. Other sources of influence included Goffman's (1968) work describing the process of institutionalization. This was influential as many of the patients had been in hospital for some time before they were admitted to the unit. Some had developed rather antisocial, institutionalized behaviour such as screaming for attention and others had not been out of doors for months. Goffman's work helped me understand why these individuals were behaving as they did and how such behaviour could be avoided.

The concept of total patient care was an important element in helping me, as the leader of a multidisciplinary team, to view each person holistically. It also helped to increase both the nursing staff's awareness of what nursing contributed to patient care and the sense of satisfaction when patients progressed.

Working in rehabilitation inspired an interest in how the body moves. I learned from other members of the multidisciplinary team but also from other sources outside the health field. In particular I found the study of contemporary dance (Murray 1979) helped me to develop an increased awareness of how my own body moved which enabled me to help patients with tasks such as learning to walk.

Rehabilitation is hard work for both the staff and the patients. It is easy to lose heart and give up when your body will not do as you wish. A working knowledge of counselling skills became very important (Egan 1994, Tschudin 1995) giving me simple frameworks for helping individuals manage their problems.

Rehabilitation also requires creativity and imagination in helping people cope with disabilities. Open University courses in humanities and a very supportive manager encouraged me to try new ideas and develop my thinking.

APPROACH TO NURSING IN AN OPERATING THEATRE SETTING

This developed out of research related to theatre work. When I began the work, my knowledge of theatre nursing was very limited and consequently I had to learn about it as I researched it.

Person

A human being who is totally dependent on nursing and medical staff for the preparation given prior to surgery, the entire surgical procedure and aftercare. Surgery is a potentially life-threatening event and the person is dependent on the skill of the professionals to ensure his/her safety.

Environment

The physical environment has two dimensions. First there is the internal environment of the person's body which will be affected by surgery and anaesthetic. The external environment comprises everything outside the person's body within the operating theatre. In addition there is the social environment which is synonymous with the culture of the theatre department. This should be one in which staff feel valued, respected and in which adverse stressors are reduced.

Health

Undergoing surgery is a stressful experience even when it is planned and wanted. Health in this context is a surgical experience for which the patient feels well prepared and from which s/he recovers successfully. Health is also a state within the operating department where tension can sometimes be very high. In this context health is part of the management of the department which should ensure that staff are not habitually required to deal with unacceptably high levels of stress.

Nursing

This is a specialized role which incorporates physical and interpersonal skills. These are used to ensure the management of the department, safety and infection control, as well as provide assistance during the surgical procedure itself. Some nurses working in this speciality become specialist practitioners which may mean that their roles overlap with those of the surgeon or anaesthetist.

Sources/influences

The major influence came from a project requiring an in depth literature review (McGee 1991). This enabled me to develop insight into the perioperative role. From there I began to investigate how theatre nurses saw their world (McGee 1993) in which patient contact is minimal since most are anaesthetized. The social environment in theatres is very important in maintaining the theatre team in a closed environment but stress can occur when lists overrun or tempers get frayed. The enclosed nature of operating theatres can make it difficult for staff to explain their difficulties to those outside on the wards thus increasing the stress.

The experience of completing the research project led me into developing a model for theatre nursing. The work of Fawcett (1995) and Wright (1990) was helpful in structuring my ideas and I also took into account the UKCC's views (UKCC 1994) on differences between working in a speciality and being a specialist practitioner (McGee 1994). The result was my first attempt to construct a formal theory of nursing.

APPROACH TO NURSING IN PAEDIATRICS

This approach grew out of discussions in class with students whilst helping them develop their views about their own practice.

Person

This has two dimensions. First of all the person is a child. The child is an individual but also part of a family group. The child is developing physically, psychologically and socially but has not yet achieved full independence. These elements of development may not all take place at the same pace. Consequently the child may be more mature in one aspect than another. The child has rights in law and is entitled to care and protection. The child is also entitled to be involved in the decision making about his/her welfare in a way that is commensurate with the individual's age and intellectual development.

The person is also the family group to which the child belongs. This may include adults who have responsibility for caring for the child – parents, grandparents, childminders, nursery staff, teachers and others.

Environment

There are several different types of environment.

(a) The child's internal environment which is both physical, psychological and emotional. This environment is growing and developing. It also affects and is affected by, the child's health.
(b) The environment includes physical settings such as home, day nursery and school. The child interacts with these environments.
(c) The family may be described as an environment in that the child lives in the family.
(d) Hospital is an environment which is particularly problematic for the child and family.

Health

This is a state in which the child receives the care and attention required for continued development towards adulthood. It is also a state in which illness and disease is managed successfully to allow the child to achieve independence. In addition health can be a state in which the family is able to function in terms of meeting the child's needs.

Nursing

The family is the first provider of care. Initially the nurse may work with the family, giving health education or specialist advice for example on feeding. The nurse provides care for the child during illness when the family is unwilling or unable to do so. This involves a range of activities and skills including manual dexterity, communication and those associated with specific elements of care. The aim of nursing is to facilitate family care when appropriate but also to recognize that the child's wishes and interests may not be the same as those of the family.

Sources/influences

Experience played a considerable part in the development of this approach alongside specialist knowledge of children with specific illnesses. Theories of child development were discussed with particular reference to their implications for providing care for children at different stages.

There was also a little cynicism. The child was seen as having rights as set out in the Children Act (1989) but the reality was that these were superseded by the wishes of adults, either as parents or professionals. Both could use their position to persuade the child to do what they thought best, which might not always be what the child wanted or needed.

The philosophy of family centred care was discussed at great length as a central element in paediatric care. In theory the family and professionals meet as equals and agree a plan of action. However, this may not always be possible if parents are unwilling to co-operate. It could even be undesirable where child protection is an issue. Professionals inevitably held more power in the relationship because of their greater knowledge and the fact that parents were to a large extent dependent on them for information, treatment and care.

These examples of beginning approaches to care represent quite different views of the central elements of nursing (Fawcett 1995). Such differences arise principally from the need to provide services to specific client groups. This in turn affects the nature of nursing and the environment in which services are delivered. Despite this, some commonalities can be identified. All three present the person as being in some way dependent on others and thus vulnerable. Nursing has a role in protecting the individual but, as the paediatric example demonstrates, this is not always achievable. Views about health are also determined in some ways by the dependence of the individual. There is a managerial element in all three examples which suggests that health is to some extent dependent on organized effort by a team of others.

The environment in all three is seen as multidimensional incorporating internal, social and physical components. Theatre nurses, however, add a unique dimension. In this field of nursing, the social environment is important because interaction with colleagues is crucial in providing some aspects of job satisfaction in a setting in which there is little chance to get to know patients. However this environment can be a source of immense stress unless managed effectively (McGee 1994).

What is most noticeable is the difference in nursing between the three examples. The activities listed, the skills and knowledge involved, reflect specific priorities either in ensuring safety (theatre nurses), promoting independence (rehabilitation nurses) or providing care in partnership with a family (paediatrics). Each form of nursing is therefore a specialized role designed to meet the needs of a specific client group. Where commonalities can be seen is in the aims of nursing which in all three examples centre on being of benefit to others, enabling them to achieve some health-related goal. Each example shows that nurses draw on a range of interpersonal, physical and management skills in order to facilitate these achievements.

It is also clear that these beginning approaches to care move beyond the philosophies found in many practice areas. These usually take a form of statements about the aims of the nursing care provided. For example, 'This ward aims to provide the highest standard of individualized care for all patients within the resources available'. Philosophies state the aims of the nursing care and as such are more like statements of intent or mission statements than an approach to care. They do not set out in any detail how such aims are to be met. The beginning approaches to care explored in this book are much broader and raise questions about how, why, when and where aims can be met.

Discussion Topic 8.1

Look at the mission statement in your practice area. What does it say? How achievable are the promises it makes? How could it be redrafted?

Discussion

IMPLEMENTING YOUR IDEAS

When you have clarified your ideas the next step is to explore ways of introducing and testing out your approach in practice. Inevitably this will involve a process of change both in your thinking and in the area where you practise. There are numerous strategies which can help you but the nursing process can also be useful in managing change as well as providing a systematic approach to nursing care.

1. Developing a nursing assessment tool

Assessment of a patient/client before surgery might include factors such as the individual's understanding of the operation and immediate post-operative period, the presence of drains, pain and intravenous infusions, fears about anaesthetic, and respiratory problems. Alternatively, assessment prior to admission to a rehabilitation unit might include a full physical assessment of the individual's capabilities; for instance whether s/he can sit unaided, feed him/herself or maintain continence. In addition it would be necessary to make some assessment of communication and comprehension abilities as well as family circumstances.

In both examples, assessment requires the collection of quite a lot of information. Look back at the summary of your approach to care and make a comprehensive list of what you think you need to know. This is the basis of your assessment tool. There are now three options open to you. You can try out the list in assessing individual patients/clients and gradually refine the tool as time goes by. Alternatively, you could use an existing assessment tool which you feel meets your needs. However this may have to be modified as it is unlikely to incorporate everything that you regard as important. Finally you could use Peplau's approach (Chapter 2) and start your assessment with a blank sheet of paper whilst keeping your list to guide you (Holt 1988). Remember that what is important is that you are able to identify problems and make an accurate nursing diagnosis.

2. Identifying the theory already in use

The official approach to care in your organization may be based on some published model such as Roper *et al.* (1990) but assessment of what is really

Table 8.1 A practitioners' model of nursing: 98 sisters/charge nurses were asked how they saw the elements of nursing with the following results:

Health is:	psychological, social and physiological well being,	46.3%
	a sense of physical and mental comfort	16.8%
Nursing is:	promoting independence,	72.6%
	an interpersonal process	16.8%
Person is:	a unique individual constantly learning and changing,	35.8%
	a whole person with basic needs	23.2%
Environment is:	external to the person	9.5%

happening may reveal a different picture. McKenna (1994) for example interviewed 98 sisters/charge nurses in 49 long stay psychiatric wards (Table 8.1) in order to try and identify their approach to nursing. In asking colleagues similar questions you will be able to identify what is important to them. For example McKenna's sample clearly saw promoting independence as an important part of their nursing but adaptation was a lesser priority.

3. Assessing your organization

An additional dimension of assessment concerns the organization in which you work. In particular there is a need to consider the following:

- Who has the power to make decisions?
- What can they make decisions about?
- Who benefits from the current situation and how?
- Who does not benefit and why?

To illustrate the issues which might arise here imagine that you are a newly appointed G grade. Several of your staff nurses have recently completed the Enrolled Nurse Conversion Course and are just beginning to adapt to their new roles. During the last few months many of the qualified staff have left and the continuity of care has rested with the health care assistants who have found themselves undertaking activities outside their normal role.

Whilst the formal authority to make decisions rests with you as the manager, actual decisions may be made by the health care assistants who may enjoy the extra responsibility. Thus they may be said to benefit from the current situation and be reluctant to give it up. On the other hand, the newly converted staff nurses are being denied the opportunity to develop their roles and thus do not benefit.

There will also be decision makers outside the nursing arena. Doctors, physiotherapists, ward clerks and other staff are all likely to be affected to some degree by changes in the nursing approach to care. These are probably people with whom you work closely anyway and on whose goodwill you rely in terms of maintaining a strong multidisciplinary team.

Consequently it is worthwhile trying to ascertain how they are likely to be affected by the introduction of your ideas so that you can present your approach in as positive a light as possible and gain their support. In the wider arena of organizational management you will have to consider other decision makers outside your immediate sphere. Unit and organizational policies may affect the way you plan to introduce your ideas. It is therefore unwise to ignore such policies, particularly if your ideas challenge the existing situation.

Finally there will be people who may be indirectly affected for example those who can make decisions about financial matters. The introduction of a new approach to nursing may incur costs and it is therefore advisable to ascertain who holds the budget and controls resources. In particular it is important to find out how best to present a case to this individual if you need to secure financial help in introducing changes.

4. Planning nursing activities

The principles of planning care will remain the same but there may be some differences in your approach now that you are using your own ideas. As your assessment technique is refined it should help you clarify priorities as you begin to plan care. A central issue here is the degree to which you are able to enter into a partnership with the patient or client and how far you have to make decisions without the full participation of the person concerned. It is the priorities of these individuals which inform the development of goals and thus personalize and individualize nursing care.

In addition to these issues, you will need to consider how best to record your priorities, goals and action plan. A model for goal setting is given in Chapter 7 which could be developed to incorporate nursing actions. What is important here is that staff can follow the documentation easily from the assessment through to the action plan.

5. Planning for your organization

The decision making pathway which helps you plan care for patients can also help you organize the introduction of your approach to nursing. You will need to summarize the findings of your assessment, identify priorities and select those which you wish to tackle first. This action plan will lead you to the construction of clear goals. These are now crucial to your success and the model set out in Chapter 7 can be used here (Table 8.2). The model allows you to set goals on an individual basis for yourself and particular colleagues. Alternatively you can set goals for groups of people. For example you might want to set up a small group to oversee and co-ordinate the introduction of your ideas rather than do all the work yourself. This group could then delegate work to other subgroups using the same goal setting model. In addition you could incorporate statements about the resources available for the achievement of each goal. This model of goal

Table 8.2 Goal setting in introducing your approach to care

Who	You (the initiator of this new approach)
will do what	will discuss new approach with medical, physiotherapy and other staff
using what means	by personal invitation to key personnel
to what degree of success	to gain their support and participation
by which date	by 21 February
Who	The steering committee
will do what	will oversee and co-ordinate
using what means	delegating specific tasks to individuals and subgroups monitoring the progress of delegated tasks and taking action if these are not achieved providing leadership for the change process addressing key management issues eg finance and staff development (statement about resources would have to be added here)
to what degree of success	whilst maintaining the delivery of nursing services
by which date	by 19 June
Who	A subgroup
will do what	will develop assessment tools
using what means	using the new approach to nursing (statement about resources to be used could also be included)
to what degree of success	for trial use with patients
by which date	by 4 March

setting therefore allows you to develop different types and levels of goal (Table 8.2).

6. Evaluating your progress

The action plan identifies tasks and priorities. The construction of clearly defined goals enables you to determine how far tasks have been achieved. First of all each goal assigns and clarifies responsibility so there can be no ambiguity about who should do what. If goals are only partially achieved or even completely unsuccessful, they can still provide a starting place for identifying the reasons for this. For example (Table 8.2) suppose that your goal for discussing your ideas with other non-nursing staff had not been successful. This could be due to a lack of key people because of vacancies or excessive workloads. Such problems may be described as structural (Donabedian 1980) because they arise as a result of a lack of resources in the organization. Alternatively, some of the meetings may not have gone as well as you had hoped. This could be due to personality differences or a lack of clarity in your ideas. Such difficulties can be described as 'process', referring to what actually happens (Donabedian 1980). Finally, even if the meetings went well it is still possible for the results or outcomes to be unsatisfactory (Donabedian 1980) perhaps because individuals have other priorities. This analysis helps to identify the source of the problem which can then be examined. It may be necessary to enlist the help of more senior staff or reconstruct the goal taking the structure, process or outcome factor into account.

Evaluation then depends on the collection and organization of information. This forms a basis for identifying the elements of success as well as failure. The next step involves decision making in which you must decide whether further action is necessary. Finally the results of the evaluation must be communicated to all those involved so that they are kept informed of developments.

SUMMARY

This chapter has outlined the factors you will need to consider in developing and implementing your own approach to nursing. In addition to clarifying your own ideas, you will need to consider the impact on the organization as a whole and identify key individuals whose support is essential. These will include your colleagues and those with decision making authority. Successful implementation of your ideas is dependent to some extent on how far you are able to negotiate with them, get them involved and even fire their enthusiasm.

Developing and introducing your own approach to nursing will take time and thought. It is perhaps best to begin in a small way, 'testing the water' (Stern 1985) to see how people will react to your ideas. Gradually you will reach a point where you can try them out, 'making a splash' (Stern 1985) sending ripples out among your colleagues and the organization. Finally you will be 'heading for shore' (Stern 1985) as your ideas become accepted and you are finally able to launch your own approach to nursing.

REFERENCES

Carper, B. (1978) Fundamental patterns of knowing in nursing. *Advances in Nursing Science* 1 (1), 13–23.

Donabedian, A. (1980) *The definitions of quality and approaches to its assessment. Explorations in quality assessment and monitoring, Vol. 1*, Health Administration Press, Ann Arbor.

Egan, G. (1994) *The skilled helper. A problem management approach to helping*, 5th edn, Brooks/Cole Publishing Co., Pacific Grove, CA.

Fawcett, J. (1995) *Analysis and evaluation of conceptual models of nursing*, 3rd edn, F.A. Davis, Philadelphia.

Goffman, I. (1968) *Asylums*, Penguin, Harmondsworth.

McGee, P. (1991) Perioperative nursing: do we need it? *British Journal of Theatre Nursing* October 1 (7), 12–17.

McGee, P. (1992) What is an advanced practitioner? *British Journal of Nursing* 1 (1), 5–6.

McGee, P. (1993) Developing a model for theatre nursing. *British Journal of Nursing* 2 (5), 262–266.

McGee, P. (1994) Rediscovering theatre nursing *British Journal of Theatre Nursing* June 4 (3), 8–10.

McKenna, H. (1994) The essential elements of a practitioners' nursing model: a survey of psychiatric nurse managers. *Journal of Advanced Nursing* 19, 870–877.

Murray, J. (1979) *Dance now. A closer look at the art of movement*, Penguin Books, Harmondsworth.

Roper, N., Logan, W. and Tierney, A. (1990) *The elements of nursing*, 3rd edn, Churchill Livingstone, Edinburgh.

Stern, P. (1985) Teaching transcultural nursing in Louisiana from the ground up. *Health Care for Women International* 6 (1–3), 175–186.

Tschudin, V. (1995) *Counselling skills for nurses*, 4th edn, Baillière Tindall, London.

United Kingdom Central Council for Nursing Midwifery and Health Visiting (1994) *The future of professional practice – the Council's standards for education and practice following registration*, UKCC, London.

Wright, S. (1990) *Building and using a model for nursing*, 2nd edn, Edward Arnold, London.

The McGee theory of nursing | 9

AN INTRODUCTION TO THE McGEE THEORY OF NURSING

This chapter draws together the main themes of the book to present a new theory of nursing together with suggestions for how this can be implemented in several different settings. The theory is based on the four elements of nursing as defined by Fawcett (1995). The influence of other theorists, particularly Peplau (1952), Henderson (1966) and Orem (1995), is acknowledged but there are a number of unique elements which reflect the real world of nursing. There are also links with earlier work on transcultural issues (McGee 1992b). The theory aims to be jargon free and reader friendly and it is hoped that readers will find it useful.

THE PERSON

The person is a human being who has several dimensions; physiological, psychological and social. Each dimension is a separate system which interacts with the other two (Fig. 9.1). In addition, the systems, and the interaction between them can be influenced by a number of factors which include *culture, ethnicity, personal preferences and heredity*. These factors may act singly or in combination. For example cultural values may influence an individual's choice of clothing but that choice may be modified by personal preferences.

The interaction between the systems and the influences upon them create a unique individual who is dynamic and constantly changing in response to demands. This individual's ability to function may be impaired by alterations in health which may occur as a result of demands made by disease, infection or accidental damage.

Physiological dimension

This is concerned with the body and body maintenance. In order to remain alive the body performs the following functions:

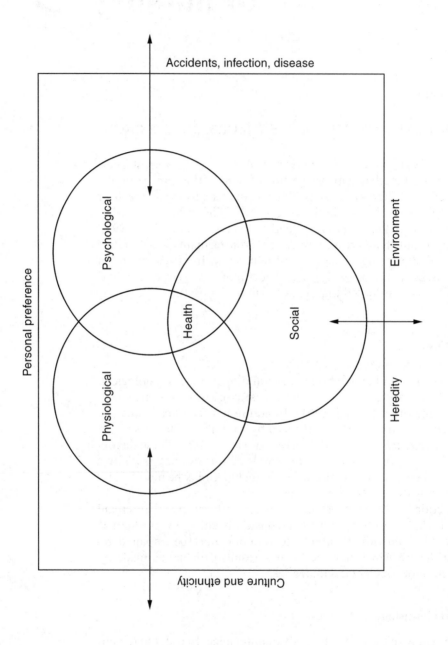

Fig. 9.1 The nature of the person.

Breathing

The body requires sufficient oxygen for cellular function and a means of excreting waste gases. Factors which may affect breathing include exercise, smoking, pollution, respiratory conditions such as asthma, infection or disease. Breathing may be affected by *heredity* in that some conditions such as asthma may run in families; by *culture* and *ethnicity* which may influence the amount of exercise and physical activity an individual undertakes, for example, in some cultures regular visits to a gymnasium may be the norm but not in others. Personal preferences may determine whether an individual engages in activities such as smoking, or working with pollutants, which are likely to affect the respiratory system. Breathing can also be affected by *disease*, for example chronic obstructive airways disease; *infection or accidental injury*.

Taking in food

The body requires food to provide energy, growth and repair of tissues and other functions. The human body requires a varied but balanced intake of carbohydrate, fats, minerals, vitamins and protein. Food is digested and absorbed through the digestive system. The preparation and intake of food is determined by *culture* in that cultural values identify which items can be eaten, how they should be prepared and cooked, how and when they should be eaten. These factors are further modified by *personal preference*, appetite and the amount of physical activity undertaken.

Within the body, the digestive system can be affected by *heredity and ethnicity* in that some conditions such as diabetes not only tend to run in families but are more common among certain ethnic groups. *Accidental injury* to the digestive system may occur as a result, for example, of alcohol abuse. *Disease*, such as Crohn's disease and infection in the intestinal system can affect both an individual's intake of food and the digestive process.

Elimination of waste products

The bowel eliminates the waste products of digestion. Problems can arise in the body when elimination is too slow (constipation) or too fast (diarrhoea). This can be due to *heredity and ethnicity* in the case of disorders such as coeliac disease which tend to be inherited and to be more prevalent among certain ethnic groups. Elimination can also be affected by acquired disease, for example, carcinoma, *infection* or *accidental damage* to the digestive system as a result of poisoning (Tortora and Anagnostakos 1990). The act of elimination itself is hedged around with values and practices arising from the individual's *culture* plus personal preferences which determine where the individual may pass faeces and what should be done afterwards.

Maintenance of fluid balance

The body requires a regular intake of fluid to maintain hydration. Fluid is excreted through the skin as sweat and through the kidneys as urine.

Culture may determine both our choice of fluids and our behaviour when we pass urine. It also affects how we care for our skin in terms of keeping clean to prevent odour and our use of clothing. These factors are further modified by *personal preferences*.

Heredity can influence fluid balance through conditions such as gout, an excessively high level of uric acid, and polycystic disease of the kidneys. In addition, acquired *diseases* such as hypertension, diabetes, renal failure or the presence of *infection* can affect the ability of body systems to maintain fluid and electrolyte balance (Tortora and Anagnostakos 1990). *Accidents* such as severe burns can cause fluid loss which also affects fluid balance.

Movement

Breathing, taking in food, excreting and maintaining water balance all involve movement. Movement is essential to meet human needs, to exercise the body and protect it from harm. In order to move, the body needs functioning skeletal, muscle and nervous systems which can be seriously affected by *disease* and *infection*. These systems can also be influenced by *heredity*. For example, osteoporosis can be an inherited condition characterized by loss of bone mass and an increased tendency to fractures. It is associated with ageing and, in terms of *ethnicity* affecting more white than black people (Tortora and Anagnostakos 1990). With regard to exercise, both *personal preferences* and *culture* may be influential in determining how much exercise an individual takes and the way in which this is undertaken. Accidents such as fractures can seriously affect the individual's ability to move.

Resting

The body needs rest and sleep on a regular basis. Lack of sleep can affect concentration and cause irritability. The presence of *infection* or *disease* can increase the individual's need for rest and sleep. There can also be an element of *personal preference* in that each individual may require a different amount of sleep. *Culture* may determine where an individual prefers to sleep and the type of bed in which that person feels most comfortable. Culture may also influence whether the whole family sleeps in the same room or whether separate rooms are used.

Growth and development

The body grows and develops throughout life from infancy to childhood, adolescence, mid-life and old age. Inherent in this aspect of the physiological dimension is the concept of maturation as the body develops throughout childhood and adolescence. In adulthood the body is able to reproduce. Further change takes place as the individual enters later life.

Growth and development are affected by endocrinal factors and *heredity*. Thus *disease* or *infection* which affect the endocrinal systems can have an effect on growth and development. An example of this is untreated underactivity in the thyroid gland which, in children, reduces both physical and intellectual development.

Growth and development are also affected by *culture* and *ethnicity* which may provide variations on what is considered the 'norm' among different groups of people. Alongside these variations is the issue of *personal preference* in that some individuals are dissatisfied with aspects of their growth and development. On one level this may be a feeling that they are either too tall or too short or that their hair is too curly/long/straight or whatever. However some individuals suffer greatly because they have not developed as expected and find, for example, that they are unable to have children.

Psychological dimension

Each individual is born into a particular family or group which provides a way of life, a culture. The individual learns the tacit aspects of the culture, the values, attitudes, beliefs alongside the more visible aspects such as how to dress and how to behave. Some, but by no means all, of the values and attitudes may be religious in origin. It is the values and attitudes generally which underpin the observable way of life that we call a culture.

Culture then not only provides a way of life but also a way of looking at the self and others through the medium of values, attitudes and beliefs which are in turn modified by the individual's personality and preferences. Thus we cannot assume that all members of a particular culture will share exactly the same opinions or live in exactly the same way.

In the context of providing patient care, culture is important in determining an individual's beliefs about health, illness, treatment and care. Successful nursing intervention will depend on identifying these factors and the ways in which they may affect outcomes. In order to achieve this, the patient must be able to communicate effectively. Communication depends on several factors which include the ability to:

- speak or convey messages in a manner which is intelligible to others;
- hear what is communicated or to receive messages in some other way and respond appropriately;
- use non-verbal signals as part of conveying and receiving messages.

In addition the individual must share a common language with those being communicated with.

Effective communication is an essential part of care and of showing respect for people. It provides a channel through which individuals can make known their perceptions of their health and their current situation. It is also essential for establishing their preferences and expectations as a basis for negotiating a care plan.

Social dimension

Each individual interacts with others through a series of multiple social roles enacted in varied settings. Primary roles (Andrews 1991) are determined by factors such as age, gender and developmental stage. Secondary roles arise from these in order to fulfil certain goals. These secondary roles are achieved positions, whereas primary roles reflect innate qualities. Examples of secondary roles include partner, parent, worker, student, householder. Tertiary roles are those additional roles which the individual chooses to take on, for example, as a member of a sports club.

Fulfilling these roles requires a wide range of social skills, among which is the ability to move smoothly from one social setting to another, changing behaviour in an appropriate way. Each setting may be based on a different way of doing things, a different culture. Thus the individual has a personal culture but must also interact with multiple cultures in the different social settings.

The individual has the right to:

- health education to maximize health potential;
- receive care when ill, from competent, professional nurses, and to know who they are;
- self-determination, autonomy, with regard to health affairs. In particular the individual has the right to be informed about his or her condition, the treatment available plus the advantages and disadvantages associated with this. The individual has the right to participate in decision making about treatment, care and discharge arrangements (Patient's Charter 1991 and 1995). The individual also has the right to decide on matters of privacy and confidentiality in terms of which members of the family and friends may have information about his or her condition;
- be treated with respect regardless of race, gender, sexual orientation, disability or any other factor which may incite discrimination.

The individual also has responsibilities. This is a rather neglected, and perhaps unfashionable, topic but one which is closely linked to that of rights and the concept of respect. Exercising one's own rights, as we have seen in the discussion about autonomy, immediately brings the individual into potential conflict with the rights of others. Negotiation is needed to create a situation in which both parties are able to exercise their rights to some extent rather than one in which one individual is always given preference over another.

In this context the individual has a responsibility to respect the rights of others. Thus others have the right to be treated with respect regardless of race, gender, sexual orientation, disability or any other factor which may incite discrimination. This includes a responsibility to treat others courteously and to avoid abusing them either verbally or physically.

Allied to this, is truth telling. Imagine that you are conducting a medicine round in a hospital ward and you say to Mrs White 'Have you any pain? Would you like something for it?' Mrs White has a responsibility to be honest with you as a nurse and answer 'Yes' or 'No' to both questions. It is not appropriate to mislead you by stating that she has no pain and does not require anything, only to complain to her family that 'I have been in agony all day and no one did anything about it'. There can be all sorts of explanations for this scenario, but the fact remains that some patients do mislead nursing staff when they have a responsibility not to do so.

Similarly, whilst the individual has the right to participate in decision making, that person has a responsibility to make his or her views and wishes known. Patients cannot expect professionals to be clairvoyant. If professionals are to stop assuming that they know best, then patients have to make some effort to participate in dialogue. Finally the individual has a responsibility to make appropriate use of health services. For example it is not appropriate to use Accident and Emergency Departments as primary care facilities, or call out a GP during the night for something which could have waited until morning.

THE NURSE

The nurse is a person, a human being, with a personal life, preferences, culture and experiences which are brought to the practice of nursing. In addition to these factors, the nurse has undergone a recognized course to achieve a statutory qualification. Thus the nurse is a professional, separate from and different to lay carers. The nurse has the same rights and responsibilities as any other human being but responsibility is increased by the professional requirements set out in the Scope of Professional Practice (UKCC 1992) and the UKCC Code of Professional Conduct (UKCC 1994).

The nurse has theoretical knowledge and a range of practical skills which facilitate the performance, for others, of those body maintenance tasks which they would otherwise do for themselves. Alternatively the nurse may teach others to perform these tasks irrespective of an individual's age, level of ability or health problems.

The nurse has a range of specialist theoretical knowledge and technical skills relevant to a specific field of practice. These may be physically, psychologically or socially orientated or a combination of all three. Whilst some of these skills, such as caring for intravenous infusions, may be transferable, others may not. The nurse must be aware of the technical skills required and keep them up to date along with the relevant knowledge base.

The nurse has well developed and regularly updated theoretical knowledge, attitudes and personal skills which facilitate day to day interaction with clients and colleagues. A central element of these is the skills required to assess, plan, implement and evaluate care. These include the knowledge and skill to teach others, through health education and promotion, and to organize care. Some nurses may choose to undertake further development of their interpersonal skills in order to perform specific roles such as counselling, specific therapeutic interventions, teaching and management.

The nurse has knowledge of local cultures and in particular has an understanding of the relationship between culture and health. The nurse has a range of skills and strategies which facilitate the application of this knowledge and understanding in a positive approach to direct, culturally appropriate, patient care.

The nurse is on a developmental journey. This lasts throughout an individual's career as that person acquires expertise and applies this to patient care. A constant factor in this journey is interacting with patients, some of whom contribute to the nurse's development.

NURSING

Nursing is a practical and interpersonal activity which enables others to improve or maintain their physiological, psychological or social health, to avoid or minimize illness or prepare for a peaceful death. The nurse can consciously adopt specific roles depending on the need of the patient at any given moment.

Physical carer

The nurse provides physical care for patients who cannot perform body maintenance tasks unaided. The nurse's intervention may be partial if the patient is able to do some tasks or complete if the patient is totally dependent.

Technician

The nurse uses technical knowledge and skills to provide, enhance or facilitate treatment. Examples of technical skills include conducting ECGs, renal dialysis and phlebotomy. However these are used only as an adjunct to nursing in order to benefit the patient and not as a replacement for the proper work of the nurse.

Specialist

The nurse has undergone post-registration education in order to develop and use an extended knowledge and skill base. This addresses a specific aspect of patient care, for example stoma care, palliative care and continence advice.

Negotiator

The nurse works with the patient to assess the current situation and identify the ways in which this has changed from what is normal for that person. This enables the nurse to determine how the patient sees the situation and what that individual sees as priorities. Nurse and patient are then able to agree a course of action which is mutually acceptable and potentially achievable.

Empowering others

The nurse enables the patient to clarify his/her perceptions, expectations and wishes with regard to treatment and care. In some instances the nurse undertakes to speak about these issues to other professionals or authority figures. However, where possible, emphasis is placed on empowering the patient to speak directly to these professionals and make his/her views known.

Teacher

The nurse provides education for the patient on matters related to body maintenance, health education, coping with illness and minimizing suffering.

Companion

The nurse, through other activities, is able to act as companion to the patient providing a source of social contact. In this context the two meet and interact as human beings rather than as patient and professional. Through this role, the nurse and the patient get to know one another and in some instances a bond can be formed between the two through which the nurse is able to provide companionship, encouragement, persuasion and support. In return the patient provides the nurse with privileged insight into the human spirit and a nobility of purpose.

Co-ordinator

The nurse acts as part of a multidisciplinary team. The nurse should know which other disciplines are contributing to the patient's care and what their specific role is. The nurse co-ordinates the interventions of these disciplines to ensure, for example, that the patient receives sufficient rest, and has time to eat.

Culture broker

The nurse ensures that care is provided in a culturally acceptable manner. Interventions may be wholly within the patient's cultural framework (cultural care preservation), promote change within that framework (cultural care accommodation) or enable the patient to cope with major change in a culturally acceptable manner (cultural care repatterning) (Leininger 1985).

HEALTH

Health is a dynamic concept which is defined by the individual and not by any external ideal. Health is feeling as well as possible – for you. Thus health can coexist with illness or a long-term condition such as diabetes. Health work is about discovering and, where possible removing, obstacles to health. These obstacles may be due to ignorance of what is needed to maintain health and may be overcome by appropriate education. However few obstacles are likely to be so easily dealt with. Health beliefs are part of a complex network of values, attitudes and beliefs which the individual assimilates as part of learning his/her culture. Health, therefore, and illness, are culturally defined and challenging health beliefs can therefore be seen as attacking the culture as a whole. Approaches must therefore be made in a culturally appropriate and sensitive manner.

Health can be affected by hereditary factors which create a predisposition to certain illnesses or conditions. In this context obstacles may not be removable and efforts need to be directed to anticipating and recognizing the onset of changes in health. Untreated or unmanaged disease presents additional obstacles which can be minimized by early intervention. Health can also be affected by other factors which are also outside the individual's control, for example, pollution and accidents. Such obstacles can be reduced through the application of safety and other strategies which reduce the risks to health.

Illness is therefore a strong possibility in all individuals' lives. It is more than a deviation from health. It is a profound change which may be temporary or permanent. It may also lead to death. Health work is also about providing care and treatment during illness and during the process of dying.

ENVIRONMENT

Each individual, patient or nurse, has an internal environment based on the physiological and psychological dimensions. These interact with one another and the social dimension to create the unique human being. The individual interacts with the external environment through the enactment of social roles which can bring about change, both in the internal environment of that person and in others. Enacting the social role of nurse, requires the individual to adopt certain values, to think and behave in certain ways in order to influence the environments of others.

The external environment is also a physical place which the individual can influence and which in turn has an effect on him/her. It is the space in which the nurse and patient meet. It is the setting in which therapeutic relationships are formed and in which care is delivered.

This concludes the overview of the McGee theory of nursing. The remainder of this chapter presents examples of the application of this theory within the framework of the nursing process. There are three scenarios. The first is based in the community and portrays a teenage boy consulting the school nurse. This is used to clarify issues to do with assessment and planning. The other two scenarios deal with an emergency situation as a patient has a myocardial infarction and the care of patient undergoing a mastectomy. These two scenarios are discussed together in order to further explore the application of the theory.

APPLICATION OF THE McGEE MODEL OF NURSING

In the following examples the McGee model is applied within the framework of the nursing process. The aim is to produce an approach to care which is simple and easy to follow.

The assessment process

When seeing a patient for the first time, the nurse must quickly identify the immediate problem or need (Fig. 9.2). Speed is essential because the presenting problem may require emergency intervention in order to save the individual's life. Alternatively, the individual may require a single nursing intervention, for example treatment for a sprained ankle, and have no further need of nursing care. In both these circumstances a full and detailed assessment is inappropriate in the short term. Later, when the emergency has resolved, or if the sprained ankle fails to heal, it may be necessary to go further. What is at issue is whether information is gathered deliberately and used for a purpose or collected and filed away to satisfy bureaucratic needs (Fig. 9.2).

The assessment process allows for more detailed exploration of a problem area. It clarifies the patient's present situation and how this has changed. It also identifies the need for assessment by a specialist. For example information about food intake may indicate the need for a detailed nutritional assessment by a specialist nurse or dietician. Example 1 shows how an assessment might be conducted using the tool shown in Fig. 9.2.

According to the school, Charlie appears to have some problem in maintaining control of his diabetes. A detailed nursing assessment shows a number of contributing factors. In the physiological dimension the disease of diabetes is very important. Charlie has had diabetes for some time and has only experienced difficulties during the current term. He is now experiencing frequent bouts of hypoglycaemia. *Personal preferences* would seem to play quite a major role in that he is choosing not to do his blood sugar monitoring and sometimes does not eat a good lunch whilst in school. The environment of the school clearly does not make any provision for people with diabetes. In addition he has began to drink alcohol which could further affect the management of his diabetes. *Heredity* is also a factor, in that there is at least one other person with this condition in his family.

In the *psychological dimension* Charlie's *culture* will be influential in his developing an adult male role. Although he seems well informed about the management of his diabetes, Charlie resents anything which sets him apart from his peers. The *social dimension* reveals that until this term he had a friend who knew about his diabetes, but presumably did not make a fuss

Identify immediate problem or need

Carry out emergency/short term intervention if required

Determine whether more detailed assessment is required

DETAILED ASSESSMENT

1. What is the current situation?

Physiological dimension

Breathing	
Food intake	
Elimination	
Fluid balance	
Movement	
Rest	
Growth and development	

Psychological dimension

Culture	
Religious beliefs	
Communication	
Perceptions of current health problems	

Social dimension

Primary roles	
Secondary roles	
Tertiary roles	

Fig. 9.2 Assessment and planning tool using the McGee theory of nursing.

2. *What is the usual situation?*

Physiological dimension

Breathing	Heredity, disease, infection, personal preferences, culture, ethnicity, accidents
Food intake	As above
Elimination	As above
Fluid balance	As above
Movement	As above
Rest	As above
Growth and development	As above

Psychological dimension

Culture	
Religious beliefs	
Communication	
Perceptions of current health problems	

Social dimension

Primary roles	
Secondary roles	
Tertiary roles	

3. *What changes can you identify?*

4. *What are the patient's expectations and how far can these be achieved?*

5. *Which nursing roles and actions would be appropriate?*

6. *Which other personnel/disciplines will be involved and what will they contribute?*

Fig. 9.2 *continued.*

about it. Charlie felt able to do his blood sugar monitoring and eat lunch at a regular time; Without this support, he feels conspicuous.

The planning process

This stage is based on negotiation which first of all takes place between the nurse and the patient. The assessment should identify the patient's perceptions of the current situation and how these could be resolved. As Example 9.1 shows, Charlie's perceptions are strongly influenced by the unwelcome attention which his diabetes attracts. The assessment also reveals unrealistic expectations in that Charlie would very much like his diabetes to go away. The first stage of planning therefore has to centre on what this patient thinks he wants and what the nurse is able to offer. Negotiating skills will help to establish some common ground between them.

Example 9.1. Assessment of a boy with diabetes in a school setting.

What is the immediate problem or need?

Charlie is a 14-year-old boy who has insulin dependent diabetes. Next term the school will be taking his class on a geography field trip which will require living away from home for five days. The teacher has already expressed reservations about taking Charlie on this trip because his diabetes seems poorly controlled. Charlie has been referred to the school nurse.

Emergency/short term intervention? not required

Is more detailed assessment required?

Yes	Why? To find out if Charlie's diabetes is unstable and the reasons for this.

DETAILED ASSESSMENT

1. What is the current situation?

Physiological dimension

Breathing	No problem
Food intake Disease Personal preference	Medical diagnosis of diabetes managed with insulin and diabetic diet. Has been experiencing hypoglycaemia with increasing frequency during this term. Feels he eats enough but sometimes, by the time he gets to the canteen, there is not much choice. If there is a queue, he buys crisps and a chocolate bar.
Elimination	No problems.

Fluid balance Disease Personal preference	No apparent problems. Is aware of the need to follow diabetic diet with regard to drinks containing sugar. Shares occasional can of lager with friends.
Movement Personal preference	Enjoys gymnastics and would like to be in the school team. Understands the need for foot care.
Rest	No problems.
Growth and development	Height 1.8 m Weight 50 kg Adolescent with some evidence of body hair; voice breaking.

Psychological dimension

Culture	Member of local, close knit family which has lived in the area for many generations. Local culture values family ties. Men and women tend to have separate roles and responsibilities.
Religious beliefs	None.
Communication	Speaks English. No problems with hearing or other senses.
Perceptions of current health problems	Resents diabetes and wants it to stop. Blood sugar monitoring attracts too much attention because the only place available to do it is the school toilets. Consequently, Charlie avoids doing blood sugar monitoring at school. He feels teacher makes too much fuss and treats him like a baby. Dislikes this. Wants to go on the field trip because everyone else is going.

Social dimension

Primary roles	Charlie is male and adolescent.
Secondary roles	Son: everything is all right at home. Brother: has three sisters, one is older than him. Friend: special friend from primary school left last term. Misses him. Has other friends but has not talked to them about his diabetes. Pupil: academically average.
Tertiary roles	Has a newspaper round Is a member of the local youth club.

2. What is the usual situation?

Food intake	Medical diagnosis at aged 8.
Disease	Occasionally unstable when ill or during periods of growth but diabetes was generally well managed until this term. Friend from primary school used to be with him when he did his blood sugar monitoring and
Personal preferences	they always went to lunch together at the same time each day.
Heredity	Aunt has diabetes.

3. What changes can you identify?

Food intake	Instability in diabetes has only been a problem this term. Has stopped doing blood sugar monitoring at school because he feels self conscious doing this where others can see him. Is not always eating a proper lunch.
Fluid balance	Has started to share the occasional lager with friends.
Growth and development	Is developing normally but is underweight.

Planning requires the nurse to identify the nursing roles and activities which may be most helpful to the patient. In example 9.1A these are likely to be *negotiator, empowering others, teacher, and culture broker*. These roles may be of direct benefit to Charlie himself but also to others in the situation.

In addition to negotiating with Charlie, the nurse may also negotiate with teaching staff regarding where blood sugar monitoring takes place and access to canteen facilities. Charlie will benefit from teaching about the importance of blood sugar monitoring, regular meals to avoid hypoglycaemia and to improve his weight. The impact of alcohol in a diabetic diet could also be included. The teachers too will find it helpful to learn about diabetes and how it should be managed. This would empower the staff, enabling them to feel more confident. Charlie will also benefit from empowerment, developing a more positive approach to his diabetes and skills in talking to others about it. Finally the nurse has to work within the context of Charlie's own way of life and the culture of the school, taking into account the ways in which things are done in that organization. The aim is cultural care accommodation (Leininger 1985) which is to help both parties adapt to the circumstances of Charlie's diabetes in a culturally appropriate manner.

Planning also requires the nurse to identify the limits of professional nursing expertise and the contributions which all members of the multidisciplinary health care team can make to patient care. These contributions need to be negotiated by the nurse and agreed with other members of the team. There may also be a need to secure the involvement of other personnel who are not health care professionals. In example 9.1A, the nurse would identify the need to involve the teaching staff, parents and possibly Charlie's GP as part of a strategy to ensure that no other cause for hypoglycaemia exists, to help prevent further episodes and to enable him to participate, successfully, in the school trip.

The successful identification of all these factors and the actions required constitute an individualized package of care which is multidisciplinary in focus and involves a range of personnel. The package must be agreed by all concerned. It should set out the actions to be taken, by whom, when and the criteria for success. The package must be delivered within an agreed timespan (Example 9.1A). These criteria form the basis for evaluation to determine the effectiveness of the package. Variations from the agreed package and the reasons for them should be noted and if necessary part or all of the package may have to be renegotiated if unforeseen circumstances arise.

Example 9.1A Planning care for Charlie.

4. What are the patient's expectations and how far can these be achieved?

> Charlie resents his diabetes and wants it to go away. This is not possible. He also wants to go on the school trip and be treated like everyone else. This is potentially achievable.

5. Which nursing roles and actions would be appropriate?

> For Charlie:
> Negotiator to establish communication channel between nurse and patient plus realistic, achievable outcomes.
>
> Teacher to revise and extend his knowledge of diabetes with particular reference to diet, blood sugar monitoring and alcohol.
>
> Empowering others to enable Charlie to develop a more positive self-image so that he is able to manage his diabetes confidently.
>
> Culture broker to provide nursing interventions in a manner which demonstrates respect for Charlie's personal culture plus the culture of the school.

> For Teachers:
> Negotiator to establish communication channel between nurse and teachers as a basis for improving facilities for Charlie and empowering staff.
>
> Teacher to inform teachers about diabetes and Charlie's needs.
>
> Empowering staff to feel more confident in dealing with Charlie and caring for him during the trip.
>
> Culture broker to provide nursing interventions in a manner which demonstrates respect for the culture of the school.

6. Which other personnel/disciplines will be involved and what will they contribute?

Parents: support and guidance in managing diabetes, help in following diabetic diet and improving weight.
GP: assessment of diabetic condition and need for any further intervention.
Teachers: providing a safe and informed environment in which Charlie can benefit from the full range of educational activities on offer.
British Diabetic Association: for advice and support plus opportunities to meet other young people with diabetes.

7. The package of care

Charlie's goal: to take part in the school trip whilst maintaining control of his diabetes.	Timescale Plan must be reviewed at end of term
Nursing : teaching for both Charlie and the staff	3 weeks
: negotiate practical solution to problem of blood sugar monitoring	1 week
: empowerment for Charlie and the staff so that they are able to talk openly about diabetes	end of term
: dietary advice and monitoring to improve weight.	3 months
Parents: support and encouragement.	continuous
GP: assessment and possibly further treatment.	1 week
Teachers: practical solution to problem of blood sugar monitoring and a safe environment for Charlie.	1 week

APPLICATION OF THE McGEE THEORY OF NURSING IN AN EMERGENCY SITUATION: ASSESSING AND PLANNING THE CARE OF A PATIENT WHO HAS EXPERIENCED A MYOCARDIAL INFARCTION

In Example 9.2 Afzal Ali has experienced a myocardial infarction. Emergency medical intervention in required before assessment can take place. In terms of the physiological dimension, this first assessment indicates the progress the patient has made so far in comparision to his condition on arrival in accident and emergency. It gives some indication of factors which may have predisposed Afzal Ali to myocardial infarction. He is for example, rather overweight (probably as a result of working long hours in a sedentary occupation), but most of the information relates to the immediate situation. This may be enough for now but as the nurse gets to know him better, a more detailed assessment reveals more relevant information about his usual lifestyle.

Example 9.2 Application of McGee's theory of nursing in an emergency situation: assessing and planning care for a patient with myocardial infarction

What is the immediate problem or need?

Afzal Ali has been brought to Accident and Emergency with severe chest pain radiating down his left arm. His blood pressure is 60/30 mmHg. His breathing is shallow and he shows signs of cyanosis.

Emergency/short term intervention?
Required.

Is more detailed assessment required?
Yes, when emergency treatment is complete.
Reason: to appraise the patient's current condition as a basis for promoting recovery from myocardial infarction.

DETAILED ASSESSMENT

1. What is the current situation?

Physiological dimension

Breathing	Airway is clear No chest pain at present Respirations: 16 per minute Oxygen in progress as prescribed No cyanosis Pulse 75 beats per minute BP 110/70 mmHg.
Food intake	Medical diagnosis of diabetes controlled by diet alone. Not able to eat at present.
Elimination	Bowels opened this morning.
Fluid balance	No oral fluids at present. IVI fluids being administered to maintain hydration. Urine output satisfactory and being monitored.
Movement	Unable to move around at present.
Rest	On bed rest.
Growth and development	Height 1.2 m Weight 85 kg Man aged 48.

Psychological dimension

Communication	Speaks some English but relies on interpreter.
Perceptions of current health problems	Very frightened by experience. Thought he would die and thinks he still might.

Social dimension

Primary roles	Middle-aged man. Father of four children.
Secondary roles	Husband: wife's name is Sahira Bibi. She does not speak English. Work role: taxi driver, works very long hours leaving little spare time.

2. What is the usual situation?

Physiological dimension

Breathing:

1. Heredity: brother died of a heart attack aged 42 years, cousin gets chest pain sometimes.
2. Personal preferences: smokes 20 cigarettes/day.
3. Culture and ethnicity: no relevant data.
4. Underlying respiratory conditions or disease: no relevant data.
5. Accidental damage to chest: no relevant data.

Food intake:

1. Heredity: history of diabetes in the family – mother, brother who died and an aunt.
2. Culture and ethnicity: Asian people have a high incidence of diabetes.
3. Personal preferences: will eat non-Asian food providing it does not contain pork/pork products which as a Moslem he is not allowed to eat.
4. Underlying conditions or disease: diabetes.
5. Accidental damage to digestive system: no relevant data.

Elimination:

1. Heredity: no relevant data.
2. Culture and ethnicity: Asian culture teaches that one hand should be used for bodily functions and the other for eating.
3. Personal preferences: prefers to use right hand only for eating.
4. Underlying conditions or disease: none.
5. Accidental damage to bowel: none.

Fluid balance:

1. Heredity: no relevant data.
2. Culture and ethnicity: no relevant data.
3. Personal preference: Enjoys coca-cola and other soft drinks.

4. Underlying conditions/disease: none.

5. Accidental damage: none.

Movement:

1. Heredity: no relevant data.

2. Culture and ethnicity: no relevant data.

3. Personal preference: does not exercise but knows that he should.

4. Underlying conditions/disease: none.

5. Accidental damage: fractured left tibia aged 19, playing cricket.

Psychological dimension

Culture	Member of Pakistani community. Values traditional way of life as it helps him to be a good Moslem. Family is very important. He is responsible for looking after his family and his parents.
Religious beliefs	Moslem. Prays five times a day. Goes to mosque on Fridays.
Communication	English is normally fairly good but uses this language mainly for work. First language is Urdu.
Perceptions of current health	Has never thought much about health but knows he is overweight. He tries to follow a reducing diet but does not find this easy. He is worried about how his wife and family will cope. He feels he has let them down. He just wants to get better and go home.

Social dimension

Secondary roles	Father: of four children aged 14, 11, 8, and 5 years.
	Son: his elderly parents live in the same house. He supports them.
Tertiary roles	None.

3. What changes can you identify?

Myocardial infarction is the biggest single change. There is a risk of re-infarction or heart failure as an additional complication. Even if he recovers this will affect his job and his ability to support the family.

4. What are the patient's expectations and how far can these be achieved?

Afzal Ali is frightened and worried that he might die. He wants to get better and go home. This is potentially achievable.

5. Which nursing roles and actions would be appropriate?

Physical carer to assist Afzal Ali whilst he is on bed rest and during the recovery phase in hospital. This will provide an opportunity for his heart to rest.
Technician to use knowledge and skills associated with cardiac monitoring and provide early intervention in the event of complications such as a cardiac arrest of heart failure.
Specialist to utilize knowledge and skill in coronary care and rehabilitation.
Negotiator to negotiate with Afzal Ali how he wishes care to be provided.
Teacher to provide education about myocardial infarction. This includes teaching about the rehabilitation phase and measures which might help prevent a recurrence. The nurse may also provide some teaching about managing a reducing diet particularly with reference to soft drinks.
Co-ordinator of the other professionals and personnel who are involved in treating and caring for Afzal Ali.
Culture broker to ensure that treatment and care are provided in a manner which shows respect for Afzal Ali's culture and religion.

6. Which other personnel/disciplines will be involved and what will they contribute?

Medicine:	specific treatment related to myocardial infarction. evaluation of progress and recovery.
Dietician:	to advise and educate about diet and soft drinks, to encourage and facilitate weight loss.
Interpreter:	to facilitate communication between Afzal Ali and members of the health care team and similarly between Sahira Bibi and the team.
Social worker:	to provide advice and help in obtaining appropriate benefits and support.

In the *physiological dimension* there is no relevant information about accidental damage or infection and there does not appear to be any evidence of underlying disease. *Heredity and ethnicity* are both factors which actively affect his health in that there is a family history of diabetes and heart disease which may be linked to lifestyle. *Culture* is also strongly linked to *personal preferences* through the medium of religious beliefs.

In the *psychological dimension* Afzal Ali clearly wishes to maintain his Moslem lifestyle and values. He has difficulty in communicating in English and so does his wife. The myocardial infarction has been a frightening experience with serious implications for his social roles. The fear of death and worry about the future could provoke another heart attack. The *social dimension* shows that he carries a lot of responsibility in supporting not only his immediate family but also his elderly parents.

Assessing a patient following myocardial infarction demonstrates the need for physical nursing care as the patient is unable to help himself. The

nurse also acts as a technician in using equipment such as cardiac monitoring, ECG machines and defibrillators to promote recovery. Allied to
this activity is the role of the specialist nurse with extended knowledge and
skill in coronary care and rehabilitation.

This application of the theory also demonstrates the needs of a patient
whose culture, and in particular his religious values, are perhaps very
different to those of many of the health professionals involved in his care.
In this context the nurse's role as culture broker is particularly important
as the aim of care is most likely to be cultural care repatterning (Leininger
1985). This will involve some major changes in lifestyle which will need to
be introduced in a culturally sensitive manner.

A number of key personnel will need to be involved. The nurse has a
role in both negotiating and co-ordinating their contributions to Afzal
Ali's treatment and care. In addition to the medical and paramedical staff,
assessment highlights the need to involve an interpreter as an integral part
of the multidisciplinary team rather than, as often happens, someone who
is peripheral to it. The interpreter has a role in facilitating communication
between the patient and all the other members of the team as well as
between them and his wife. This role is especially important as the nurse is
unable to act as companion. Unless the nurse shares the patient's language
or has an interpreter present, communication will be severely curtailed.
Non-verbal signals could be used but there is a possibility that these may
be interpreted differently across cultural divides.

APPLICATION OF THE McGEE THEORY OF NURSING IN ASSESSING AND PLANNING THE CARE OF A PATIENT UNDERGOING SURGERY

In Example 9.3 Freda Smith is admitted to hospital for a mastectomy. On
admission the assessment shows few problems other those directly related
to the reason for admission. As the nurse gets to know Freda Smith further
information can be obtained. In the *physiological dimension* she appears to
be very healthy with little influence from any factors. In the *psychological
dimension* she is clearly worried about her children rather than herself and
seems not to be aware of the possibility of future treatment. In the *social
dimension* she is carrying a lot of responsibility in multiple social roles both
as a single parent and in helping to look after her brother.

**Example 9.3 Application of the McGee model of nursing in the care of a patient
undergoing surgery. Assessing and planning care for a patient undergoing mastectomy.**

What is the immediate problem or need?

> Freda Smith is admitted to hospital for a mastectomy following a diagnosis of
> carcinoma in her right breast.

Emergency/short term intervention?
Not required.

Is more detailed assessment required?
Yes
Reason: to identify factors which may affect post-operative recovery and future treatment.

DETAILED ASSESSMENT

1. What is the current situation?

Physiological dimension

Breathing	No problems.
Food intake	No problems.
Elimination	No problems.
Fluid balance	No problems with drinking fluids. Has experienced stress incontinence since the birth of her last child 10 years ago.
Movement	No problems.
Rest	Finds it difficult to sleep.
Growth and development	Height 1.7 m. Weight 60 kg 36-year-old woman with two children. Has lump in right breast.

Psychological dimension

Communication	Speaks English. No difficulties with sight or hearing.
Perceptions of current health problem	Was expecting the diagnosis after finding the lump in her breast.

Social dimension

Primary roles	Freda Smith is a young woman with two children.
Secondary roles	Mother: children are aged 10 and 13 years. She has arranged for them to be cared for by their grandparents whilst she is in hospital.

2. What is the usual situation?

Breathing:
1. Heredity: no relevant data
2. Personal preferences: does not smoke

3. Culture and ethnicity: no relevant data

4. Underlying respiratory conditions or disease: none but worked with asbestos for 6 months, 15 years ago.

5. Accidental damage to chest: none

Food intake:

1. Heredity: no relevant data

2. Culture and ethnicity: no relevant data

3. Personal preferences: vegetarian

4. Underlying conditions or disease: none

5. Accidental damage to digestive system: no relevant data

Elimination:

1. Heredity: no relevant data

2. Culture and ethnicity: no relevant data

3. Personal preferences: none

4. Underlying conditions or disease: none

5. Accidental damage to bowel: none

Fluid balance:

1. Heredity: no relevant data

2. Culture and ethnicity: no relevant data

3. Personal preference: prefers herbal teas and decaffeinated drinks

4. Underlying conditions/disease: none

5. Accidental damage: none

Movement

1. Heredity: no relevant data

2. Culture and ethnicity: no relevant data

3. Personal preference: works out every week and walks everywhere

4. Underlying conditions/disease: none

5. Accidental damage: none

Rest

1. Heredity: no relevant data

2. Culture and ethnicity: no relevant data

3. Personal preference: normally sleeps well

4. Underlying conditions/disease: none

5. Accidental damage: none

Growth and development
Menstruating every month and has been using oral contraceptives.

SUMMARY

This chapter has drawn together many of the themes discussed earlier in the book. These have been used to form the foundation of the McGee theory of nursing. This theory has been influenced by the work of Peplau, Orem and Henderson but contributes some unique perspectives in considering nursing roles and the concept of the nurse as a person.

This chapter has also provided worked examples of the ways in which this theory of nursing can be applied to the assessment of patients and the planning of their care. It demonstrates that the theory can be used with patients who have very different needs both in hospital and elsewhere.

REFERENCES

Andrews, H. A. (1991) *Overview of the role function mode. Cited in:* Roy, C. and Andrews, H. A., *The Roy adaptation model: the definitive statement*, Norwalk, Connecticut, Appleton and Lange.
Department of Health (1991) *The Patient's Charter*, DOH, London.
Department of Health (1995) *The Patient's Charter and You*, DOH, London.
Fawcett, J. (1995) *Analysis and evaluation of conceptual models of nursing*, FA Davis, Philadelphia.
Henderson, V. (1966) *The nature of nursing*, Macmillan, New York.
National Health Service Executive (1995) *The Patient's Charter*, 2nd edn, NHSE, Leeds.
Leininger, M. (1985) Transcultural nursing diversity and universality: a theory of nursing. *Nursing and health care*, 6 (4), 209–212.
McGee, P. (1992b) *Teaching transcultural care: a guide for teachers of nursing and health care*, Chapman and Hall, London.
Orem, D. (1995) *Nursing, concepts and practices*, 5th edn, CV Mosby, St Louis.
Peplau, H. (1952) *Interpersonal relations in nursing*, GP Putnam, New York.
Tortora and Anagnostakos (1990) *Principles of anatomy and physiology*, 6th edn, Harper and Row, New York.
United Kingdom Central Council for Nursing Midwifery and Health Visiting (1992) *The scope of professional practice*, UKCC, London.
United Kingdom Central Council for Nursing Midwifery and Health Visiting (1984) *Code of professional conduct*, UKCC, London.

Index

Page numbers in **bold** refer to figures; page numbers in *italic* refer to tables.